understanding Nutrition

by

Dr Clemency Mitchell

Dr Clemency Mitchell has had 30 years in general medical practice, even longer teaching college students health principles, running health, nutrition and cookery courses. She cooks at home for a household varying from two to a dozen or more.

'My years in general practice taught me that a change in diet and lifestyle would be by far the best prescription for most chronic health problems,' writes Dr Mitchell. 'As a teacher I have had the opportunity to study nutrition and other health-related topics in more detail than most medical doctors are able to.'

Dr Mitchell lives in Berkshire with her husband Dr Colin Mitchell (author of *Origins, Accident or Design?*). They have four children and nine grandchildren.

Disclaimer

Although diet and nutrition are crucial to the maintenance and recovery of health, people can become ill even on the most perfect diet. The information in this book can have a very positive impact on your health, but it should not take the place of appropriate medical advice. It is usually best to make dietary changes gradually, and if you have medical problems and are on medication, it is very important to discuss any major changes you plan to make with your doctor or other health advisor.

First published in 2011
Copyright © 2011

Design and layout: Steve Holden & Abigail Murphy

British Library Cataloguing in Publication Data. A catalogue record for this book is available from the British Library.

ISBN 978-1-904685-55-5

Published by
The Stanborough Press Limited
Alma Park, Grantham, Lincs.

Printed in China

understanding Nutrition

by

Dr Clemency Mitchell

Contents

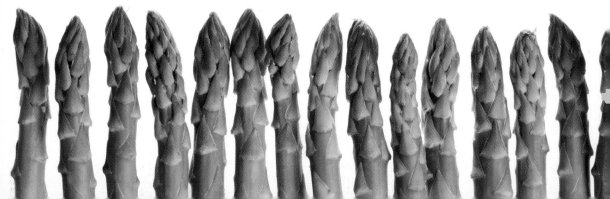

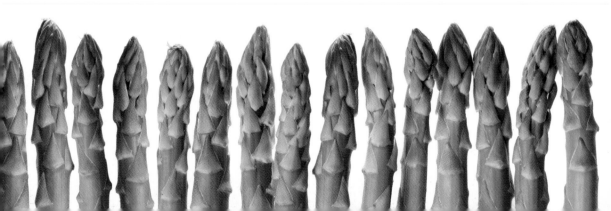

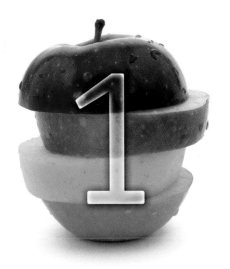

General introduction

Invest in your health!

This is one of the best investments anyone can possibly make. It is an investment that does not demand much in the way of capital outlay and, although the full benefits are in the future, it starts to pay dividends right away.

The downside of living longer

Nowadays, the average woman in the West can expect to live for about eighty years, and the average man for seventy-five, several years more than thirty or forty years ago. But there is a downside to living longer in the comfortable Western world: the ill health and disability that mar the final years of these long lives. Here the average person can expect to spend the last seven or eight years of his life suffering from chronic degenerative problems, ranging from high blood pressure with its threat of heart disease and stroke, to crippling osteoarthritis, with its long and painful wait for hip or knee replacement surgery.

It's a pity that so many people wait until they are old to think about investing in health, because, as with financial investments, the sooner they start the scheme, the greater the benefit. But, even after a lifetime of neglect, improving lifestyle still pays valuable dividends.

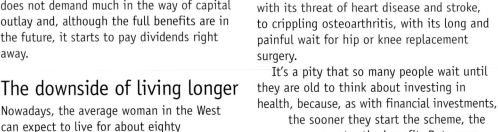

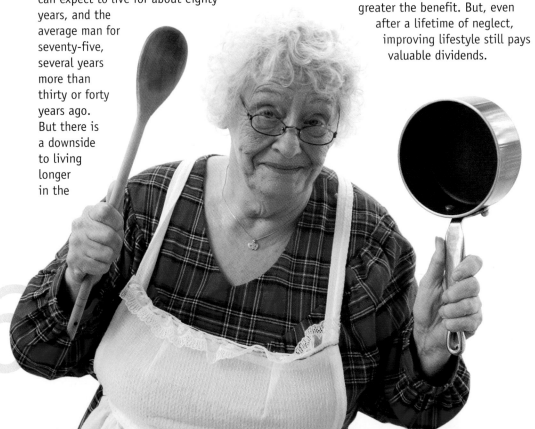

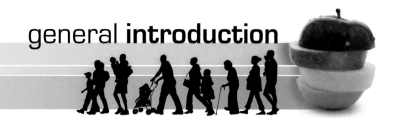

The obesity epidemic

A few years ago the UK had the distinction of being named as the fattest nation in Europe, and since then there have been constant reminders in the media that being a nation of fatties carries a high price in terms of chronic disease. Obesity is a major factor in almost all the degenerative diseases: diabetes, heart disease, cancer, arthritis – problems that shorten life or seriously interfere with its quality. At the same time, because we admire slimness, we have an epidemic of eating disorders.

Worldwide problems

These are no longer just problems of the rich countries of the West, with their abundance of rich food and sedentary lifestyles. Problems of nutrition occur in all societies. In half the world the main problem is to get enough to eat. For the other half the problem is to persuade people to choose the right food. The obesity epidemic is worldwide, and wherever people adopt the unhealthy features of the Western lifestyle there are problems. In many countries the degenerative diseases of the rich, developed countries exist side by side with the infectious diseases and malnutrition of poverty.

Lifestyle is the key

How long we live and how healthy we are both depend on what we eat, how much exercise we get, the poisons we take into our bodies, our frame of mind, and the one we cannot change, our genes. The last one explains why a healthy lifestyle doesn't guarantee a long and healthy life. We cannot change the genes we inherit from our parents, but, contrary to popular opinion, apart from certain rare inherited diseases, lifestyle is more important than genetic inheritance. We cannot change our past history either, but we can do plenty of things to help undo the effects of our past mistakes. Our bodies are so well designed that they have inbuilt corrective and healing properties, and, as soon as conditions are put right, healing begins. This is true of smoking, alcohol, faulty diet and lack of exercise, to name a few. A healthy lifestyle can at best prevent or at least postpone degenerative disease. As doctors who have wide experience of lifestyle medicine say: Genes load the gun: lifestyle pulls the trigger.

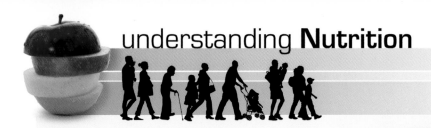

Four keys to understanding the importance of nutrition

- **Good food** is the foundation for good health at all ages.
A good diet from pregnancy and childhood onwards leads to a long and healthy life.

- **Too little food** in pregnancy and childhood results in poor growth and lasting disabilities. Too little food at all ages leads to deficiency diseases and low resistance to infections of all sorts, including life-threatening ones like TB, malaria and AIDS.

- **Deficient food** – where there are enough calories but not enough micronutrients – in pregnancy and childhood sets the scene for degenerative disease in adult life.

- **Excess food** in the form of too many calories from fat and sugar-rich, refined foods, with their micronutrient deficiencies, at any age, sets people up for all the life-shortening degenerative conditions, including diabetes, heart disease, stroke and cancer.

Good food has healing properties that help to restore health and undo the effects of previous poor diets.

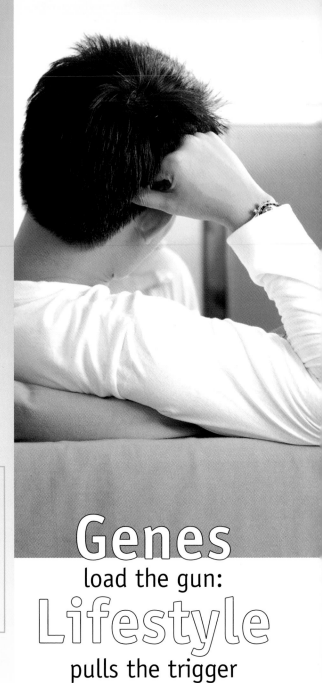

Genes load the gun: **Lifestyle** pulls the trigger

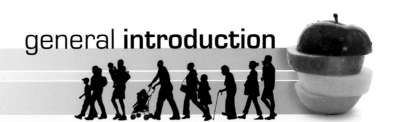

Obesity is defined as the state of being 20% or more above one's recommended weight.

Recommended weights are calculated from long-term studies of medical records that include height, weight, medical history, age and cause of death.

Lifestyle includes what we take into our bodies and how we use them. What we take into our bodies includes all we eat and drink or smoke, and all drugs, whether medicinal or recreational, and even the air we breathe. How we use our bodies involves all our physical activities, including how we exercise and rest. Lifestyle also includes what we take into our minds and how we use them.

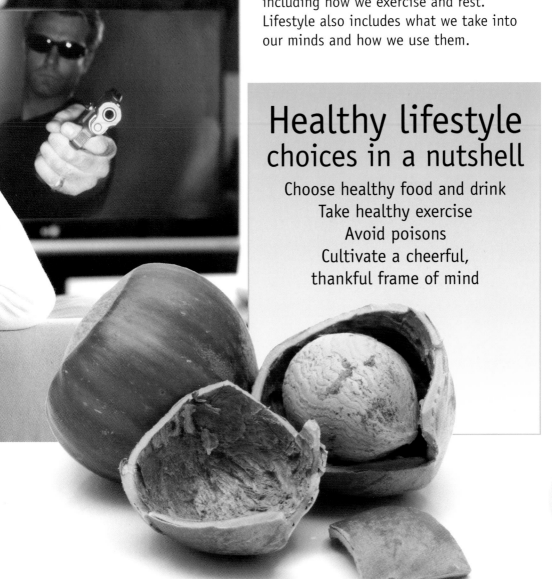

Healthy lifestyle
choices in a nutshell
Choose healthy food and drink
Take healthy exercise
Avoid poisons
Cultivate a cheerful,
thankful frame of mind

9

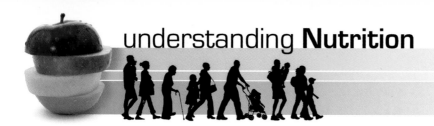

understanding **Nutrition**

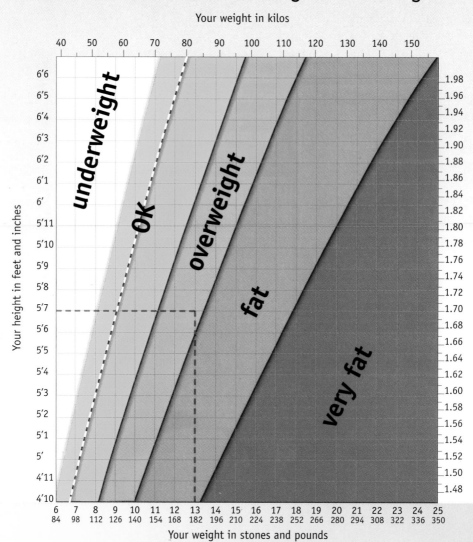

Table of recommended heights and weights

Your weight in kilos

Your height in feet and inches

Your height in metres

underweight

OK

overweight

fat

very fat

Your weight in stones and pounds

Source: www.eatwell.gov.uk/healthydiet/healthyweight/heightweightchart

10

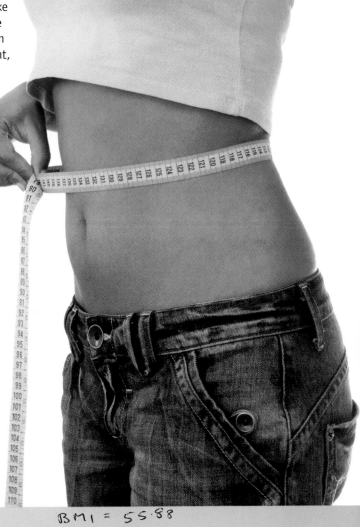

Height-weight charts are good general guides but do not always give the correct picture, because they don't take account of muscle and bone mass. The well-developed muscles of a sportsman may make him appear to be overweight, while the small muscles and thinner bones of an elderly person may hide the fact that they are carrying too much fat.

Body Mass Index (BMI) is a frequently used measurement of body weight in proportion to height for adults. It is calculated by dividing the weight in kilos by the height in metres squared, but it also has its limitations, and for the elderly, waist-hip ratio is more useful.

Waist-hip Ratio (WHR). Neither height-weight charts nor BMI indicates where the main fat stores are, and this can be important because excess fat stored in the abdomen (the 'apple-shaped' person) carries a higher risk of heart disease, stroke and diabetes than does fat stored more evenly throughout the body, including the hips (the 'pear-shaped' person). A quick check can be made by measuring the waist-hip ratio: simply measure the waist (at what should be the narrowest part of the abdomen, just above the umbilicus) and the hips at their widest point. Divide the waist by the hips to get the ratio. Over 0.8 for a woman and 9.5 for a man spell danger.

BMI = 55.88
WHR = 0.9

11

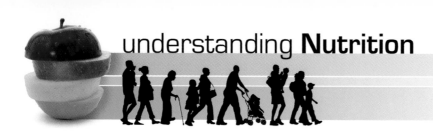

Making choices

Scientific advance and hi-tech medical care enable people in the countries where it's available to prolong their lives, but often only for a few years of increasing disability. Hi-tech medicine is lifesaving in trauma and other emergencies, but it is more involved in fighting than in preventing chronic degenerative disease. It is also very expensive in both equipment and manpower. Even the richest countries struggle to provide medical care for the epidemic of degenerative disease they face. Governments and health institutions have a huge task ahead.

Prevention is still much better than cure, and it is something that anyone old enough to understand the issues can do something about.

Food and eating habits

Some of our most important health choices are to do with what we eat and drink. Getting the maximum benefit from our food depends not only on choosing the right food, but also when to eat it, how much of it to eat and our state of mind when we eat it.

As well as a simple introduction to the principles of nutrition, this book has information about nutrition's place in the prevention and healing of disease. There are sections on keeping your digestive system healthy and practical advice about meal planning and cooking.

Other lifestyle factors are important, too. Diet isn't everything, so there is a small section about exercise and one about motivation for lasting changes in lifestyle and eating habits.

12

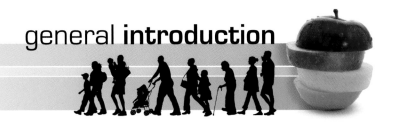

Nutrition overview

Macronutrients

The BIG nutrients are the ones we take in visible quantities. They are **protein**, **carbohydrate** and **fat**, the fuel, building and maintenance foods. We need them in the right proportions for our own particular needs, depending on our age, gender, occupation, state of health, and even the climate we live in.

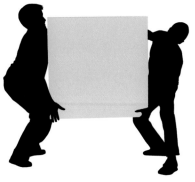

We need food for energy. It's the fuel our bodies burn to provide the energy for all our activities, and all our body's complex biochemical processes. Food energy is

measured in calories. High calorie food is high-energy food. This is what we need for strenuous manual work or sport, but not what we need if we spend most of our work and leisure sitting down in a warm and comfortable environment.

13

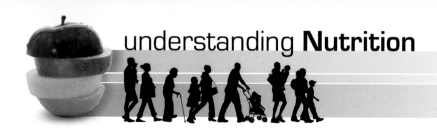

Micronutrients

Although micronutrients come in tiny
amounts and are usually invisible, they are
just as important as the macronutrients. They
do not provide fuel or building materials, but
they have vitally important roles in all the
body's complex systems for growth,
reproduction, maintenance and healing. There
are three main groups of micronutrients:
vitamins, minerals and phytochemicals.

Vitamins were discovered when they were
found to cure deficiency diseases. The
vitamin industry was born, and although
many people on poor diets have benefited
from supplements, many others have wasted
a great deal of money on taking pills instead
of eating good food.

Minerals came into prominence long ago
when it was realised that anaemia could be
helped by iron, and that calcium was
necessary for healthy bones. Mineral
supplements have helped many people, but
the mineral mega-businesses have
also persuaded many people to
spend a great deal of money
on supplements that they
do not need.

Phytochemicals have been in the news for
much less time, and came into prominence
when the epidemiologists discovered that the
more plant foods in the diet, the less cancer.
The first case to become well known was that
of the brassica plants – the cabbage family.
Scientists found an inverse relationship
between brassica plants in the diet and
cancer incidence, so the plants were studied
to discover just what the active health-
promoting substances were. These
substances, which occur in minute amounts,
and only in plants, are the phytochemicals.
(The name simply means 'plant chemicals'.)
There are many thousands of them, with
different chemical structures and different
functions.

Micronutrients are an exciting area to
study. They are the subject of intense
research, as microbiologists probe more
deeply into the incredibly complex biological
structures and functions of animals and
plants. We can be sure that in the next few
years much more will be known about
the amazing
interactions
of foods and
the human
body.

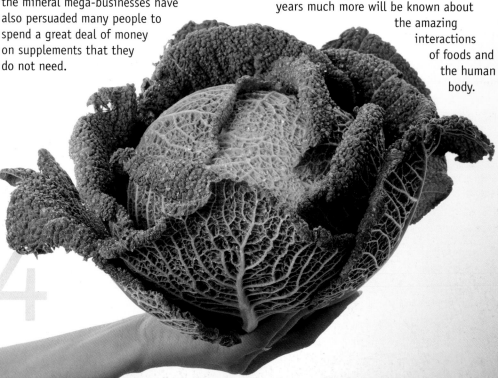

Water – the top priority nutrient

Although water is not usually thought of as a nutrient, it has a very important place in nutrition. The adult human body is 60-70% water. The brain is 85% water. All our body's activities depend on water. The blood that transports nutrients and waste products is mainly water, and all our cells contain water and are surrounded by water. Water is needed for metabolism, temperature control, as a lubricant and shock absorber, and for many other functions. The water balance is so important that we can live only for a few days without water, whereas shortages of other nutrients can take weeks, months or even years to develop.

Almost all foods contain water. Fruit and vegetables in their fresh and natural state have the highest water content. This is by design, and its function is to give a sense of fullness and satisfaction after eating them, and also to help maintain our water input. One of the problems with refined foods is that, as well as lacking fibre they also lack water, which makes them more concentrated and less filling.

Recommendations for water intake vary from one to two litres a day, with more in hot weather or when one is exercising strenuously. Good hydration has many bonuses. It boosts the immune system, thereby helping it to resist infections. It thins the blood, lowering the blood pressure and helping to prevent heart attacks, strokes and blood clots. It also helps to relieve headaches and many muscular aches and pains. A good rule of thumb is to drink enough to keep the urine pale and clear. In practical terms, this will work out to several large glasses of water a day for most people in temperate climate conditions. A good way to start the day is to take a large drink of water on rising, say a pint (a generous half litre), and then take mid-morning, mid-afternoon and mid-evening drinks. It is better not to drink very much with meals, as the fluids dilute the digestive juices and slow down the digestive process.

15

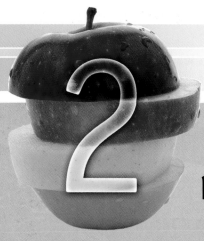

2 The macronutrients

The carbohydrates (CHOs)

There are two digestible types of carbohydrates, the **starches** and **sugars**, and one indigestible type, **fibre**. The name 'carbohydrate' indicates that these foods are made from carbon and water. Plants use the sun's energy to build them up from carbon dioxide in the atmosphere and water from the ground. They are the plants' main energy store, and they are the body's preferred source of fuel to provide the energy for all its activities.

The plants initially form simple sugar molecules, which they can build into long complex chains of starch, as in cereals, or keep as simple sugars in fruits. In addition, some are built into long, indigestible chains of fibre. When we eat them, the digestible carbohydrates get broken down to single sugar molecules which the blood transports, via the liver, to the tissue cells. There they react with oxygen to produce energy, water and carbon dioxide. It's a very clean and efficient process, with no harmful waste products. Carbohydrates are the body's premium fuel, and should be its main source of energy.

Sugars come in two forms, single sugar units (monosaccharides) and double sugar units (disaccharides).

Monosaccharides are single sugar molecules, glucose and fructose being the most important ones. All the other CHOs are made up from these sugar units linked together.

Glucose is very important in human nutrition. Starches are almost exclusively made of glucose molecules and the important disaccharides contain glucose. Glucose is the form in which sugar is transported in the blood to the tissues, where it provides the fuel for their activities. As it is a simple sugar molecule, it does not need to be digested before it is absorbed into the bloodstream, which is why glucose is viewed as a source of instant energy.

Fructose is the main sugar in fruit, slightly sweeter than glucose, and equally quickly absorbed.

Galactose is one of the sugars in milk.

Disaccharides are also simple sugars, formed by linking two monosaccharides together. The digestive system quickly breaks them down and they can enter the bloodstream almost as quickly as glucose. The most important ones are sucrose, maltose and lactose. *Sucrose* is our everyday table sugar. It is formed from one molecule each of glucose and fructose linked together. The main sources of sucrose are sugar cane and sugar beet.

Lactose is another milk sugar, so is found in all dairy produce.

Maltose is the main constituent of malt, a sweet sticky brown liquid, rich in B vitamins. It is used in the food industry in malted breakfast cereals and in malted milk drinks. Maltose is a stage in the digestion of starch that is formed when grains are sprouted, and it is important in brewing.

In their natural state, sugars from plants come packaged with large amounts of fibre. Sugar cane is so fibrous that you need a yard of it to get a teaspoonful of sugar. Sugar beets are also very fibrous. The processing of sugar involves removing the fibre and concentrating the sugar into a dark, treacly liquid, which can then be refined to the pure white crystals of granulated table sugar.

Starch is the main form of carbohydrate storage in plants, and it is the main source of food energy for most of the world's population – rice in Asia, wheat in Europe and North America, maize in Central and South America, millet, yams and cassava in Africa, rye and barley elsewhere. These cereals are not only the ideal sources of food energy; they are very valuable economically, as it takes far less land to produce these foods than it does to produce meat or other animal products.

These complex carbohydrates are long chains of hundreds of simple sugar molecules linked together. They take longer to digest than the sugars and therefore do not push up the blood sugar level as quickly. The naturally high fibre content of unrefined starchy foods helps keep the supply of energy steady all day. At the same time, the fibre gives a feeling of fullness and satisfaction that discourages overeating.

17

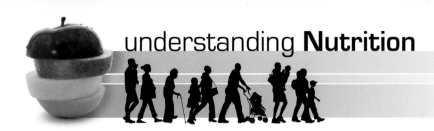

The digestion of carbohydrates

Refined **sugars** like sucrose and concentrated sugars like malt, honey and the sugars in fruit juices are very rapidly broken down and absorbed. When there is no fibre, they can enter the bloodstream within minutes. This produces a quick rise in blood sugar, resulting in a quick energy boost – a sugar high. But the high is only temporary, because the pancreas reacts to the high blood sugar level by sending out a surge of insulin which gets the sugar molecules out of the bloodstream and into the cells. This brings the blood sugar down to safe levels, but, especially if there is no fibre, may lower it so fast that it causes feelings of weakness, hunger and shakiness. A sugary snack may give instant but temporary relief. In whole plant foods the sugar is packaged with fibre which slows the digestion and absorption, and allows the sugar to enter the bloodstream more slowly, putting less stress on the pancreas. Eating an apple or banana would be better, as the fibre in these foods slows the absorption of sugar, so one feels satisfied for longer.

Starches, in their long chains, break down more slowly, a process starting in the mouth, with an enzyme in the saliva (note how a piece of plain bread gets sweeter as you chew it). Chewing well gets starch digestion off to a good start. When the process is completed, the small intestine and the sugar molecules are absorbed from there and taken to the liver on their way to the general circulation. The fibre content of *unrefined* starches slows their digestion even more. This longer digestion process keeps the blood sugar level steady, avoiding the problems of both high and low blood sugar.

Some glucose is stored in the liver and muscles as glycogen, the body's short-term energy store. These are large multi-branched starch-like molecules that can rapidly be broken down to provide glucose whenever it is needed. Excess glucose is stored as fat, the body's long-term energy store.

What about the natural sugar in fruits?

The fibre present in whole fruits slows down the release of sugar to the bloodstream, and also discourages overeating. Fruit juices, though unrefined, have lost their fibre, and so are concentrated sugars, and that for some people can cause the same problems as foods high in refined sugar. Most people can eat plenty of fruit in its natural state without having to worry about their blood sugar.

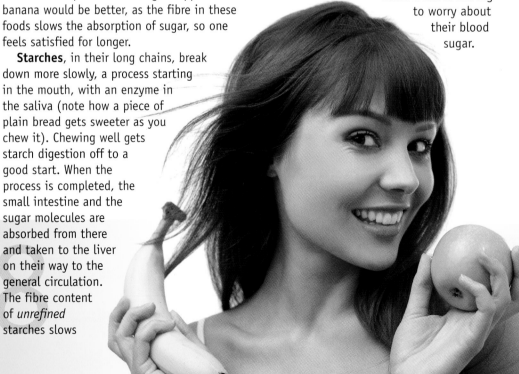

18

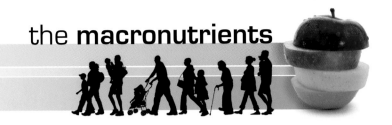
The blood sugar level must be

regulated very carefully, as a constant supply of glucose is needed for the brain. If it is too low, the brain cannot function properly; if it is too high, tissues are damaged. Blood sugar levels are regulated by two hormones, **insulin** and **glucagon**. After a meal, the blood sugar rises and the pancreas sends insulin into the bloodstream with the effect of moving the sugar out of the blood and into the cells to do its work. When the blood sugar gets low, glucagon appears on the scene to release sugar back into the circulation to ensure that there is enough for the brain to keep going.

Simple sugars have the advantage of being very rapidly absorbed for emergency energy supplies, but if large amounts are eaten, they can raise the blood sugar level too quickly. Insulin is then produced to get the excess sugar into the cells. The slow absorption of the sugar molecules from the breakdown of the starches gives a much longer lasting feeling of satisfaction after the meal, and

maintains a much more stable blood sugar level. The ideal is to base meals on the complex carbohydrates, add plenty of fruit or vegetables, and limit the use of refined sugar, for the reasons below.

The sour side of refined sugar

Tooth decay. Too much sugar is very harmful to the teeth, especially children's teeth, and especially if it is in frequent or prolonged contact with the teeth. Sweets and biscuits between meals and the frequent use of sugary soft drinks cause major problems.

White blood cells. Sugar-rich foods have been shown to depress the activity of the white blood cells that fight infections. Research at the Loma Linda School of Dentistry showed that a double sized banana split could reduce the number of bacteria a white blood cell could deal with from fourteen to one. This helps to explain the sugar-and-tooth-decay connection, and why frequent skin infections can be the first signs of diabetes.

The **Glycaemic Index** or GI is a measure of the effects of carbohydrate foods on blood sugar levels. It indicates how quickly the sugar they contain is absorbed into the bloodstream. Foods that are rapidly digested and absorbed have a high GI and they can cause marked fluctuations in blood sugar levels. Foods that are slowly digested and absorbed have a low GI and produce a gradual rise in blood sugar. Low GI diets have proven health benefits, especially for people with diabetes. They improve blood levels of both sugar and lipids, including cholesterol, in people with diabetes. They also help with weight control, because they are more satisfying and so help to control appetite and delay hunger.

So how do we know what to eat? Working out the GI levels of one's diet could be as complex and tedious as counting calories, but it doesn't have to be. In general, the refined carbohydrates, white bread, bagels, croissants, cakes, biscuits and so on, are the high GI foods; whole foods – whole-wheat flour and other unrefined starches – are low GI foods. There are some exceptions, but the natural unrefined plant-food diet will have the lowest GI, and another piece of good news: low GI foods will slow down the digestion of high GI foods, so lowering the GI level of the whole meal.

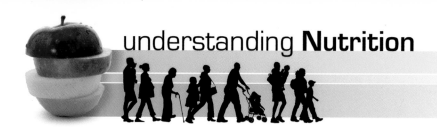

Empty calories. Refined sugar comes with no extras – no micronutrients and no fibre, as they have all been removed in the refining process – just empty calories. The real danger of empty calorie foods is that they displace nutritious food in the diet. Filling up on junk food just does not leave room for the fruits, vegetables and whole grains that we need to supply the micronutrients. Eating many empty calories means missing out on those important things.

Overweight and obesity. In the West most sugar is eaten in the refined form. Having lost all its vitamins, minerals and fibre, it is neither filling nor satisfying. The sugar-eater needs those missing nutrients, but interprets the dissatisfaction as a need for more sugar, eats more empty calories, and those extra calories are stored as fat.

Diabetes. Too much sugar along with too much fat can lead to diabetes, where the sugar builds up in the blood instead of going into the cells where it is needed. The high blood sugar levels in untreated diabetes damage all sorts of tissues, including the kidneys, heart and blood vessels, and the lens and retina of the eye. Unfortunately, many older people do not realise that they are diabetic until the damage has begun. Part of the solution – avoid refined sugar.

The benefits of unrefined starch

Slower digestion and slower glucose release. This is partly because the starch molecules are very large and take longer to digest, but even more important is the fibre that comes with the unrefined starches, and slows the process even more. This slow digestion and absorption keeps the blood sugar levels steady and spares the pancreas from having to provide so much insulin.

More vitamins, minerals and phytochemicals. The darker parts of cereal grains contain most of the fibre and much of the mineral, vitamin and phytochemical content. These are lost when the grains are refined.

Vitamins – especially of the B complex group. Unrefined grains are one of the best sources of these vitamins that are vital for the proper function of the brain and nervous system.

Minerals – especially iron and calcium. The dark colours of the outer layers contain iron, and there is a legal requirement to return some of these things back to white flour.

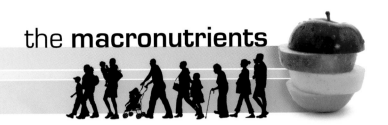

Carbohydrates and weight control

One gram of fat produces nine calories, while one gram of carbohydrate produces only four. Unrefined starches are filling and are an aid to weight control. Refined carbohydrates, like white sugar, have lost all their fibre, are not filling, and make it easy to take in too many calories. As well as fibre, other essential nutrients are lost, and this lack drives one to eat more empty calories.

Are starchy foods fattening?

Fat is the most fattening food. One gram of fat produces nine calories, while one gram of carbohydrate produces only four. The problems are caused by refining carbohydrate foods. With the fibre removed, the foods are less filling, less satisfying, and it is easy to overeat, which, in turn, makes you fat. (Essential vitamins and minerals are also lost in refining.) And, of course, there is the fat that you choose to add to the starchy food – it is not the bread that makes you fat but the butter, jam or cheese you may eat with it.

Practical steps to the right weight

Unrefined starches in their natural form, such as baked potatoes, brown rice and whole-wheat bread, fill us up without overloading our systems with calories. Whole fruit, with its full complement of fibre, has the same effect. Add a variety of vegetables and fruits, some of them raw, and some nuts and seeds, and you will have a very healthy diet. You can eat more food and still lose weight. You will have more consistent energy levels and greater endurance. Your arteries will also be kept clean!

What more could you wish?

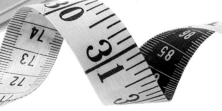

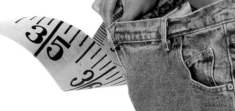

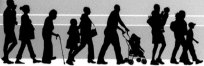

Biochemistry note

CHOs are produced in plants. They use the sun's energy to transform **carbon dioxide** from the air and water from the ground into simple sugar molecules.

ENERGY + WATER + CARBON DIOXIDE = SUGAR

Some of these sugar molecules are built into starch chains by enzymes, which link them together by removing water molecules. When starch is eaten, enzymes in the digestive tract do the reverse, adding water molecules back to split the links. The simple sugar molecules are absorbed into the blood and taken to the liver for sorting, before being transported in the general circulation to the body's trillions of cells, which use them as fuel by burning them with oxygen to produce energy and the by-products, carbon dioxide and water.

SUGAR + OXYGEN = ENERGY + WATER + CARBON DIOXIDE

Any extra is converted to glycogen for short-term storage
or to fat for long-term storage.

Focus on fibre

Fibre includes a variety of substances that form the texture and framework of plants. Unlike the digestive system of many animals, ours do not have the enzymes to digest them, so they pass through our digestive tracts and do not provide us with any nutrition. Because fibre is not digested, in the past people thought of it as useless roughage, but now we know that it is extremely important and helps to protect us against many diseases. Fibre is found in all natural plant foods, and, although there are several different types, for practical purposes they come in two main groups, according to whether or not they are soluble in water. Most plants will have a mixture of different fibres, with one predominating. The insoluble fibres are mainly in the cereals, the soluble in fruits. Nuts and legumes are also high in fibre and have a mixture of both kinds. Cereals are the main source of fibre in most diets. Unrefined cereals provide an abundance; refined cereals are deficient, having lost most of the fibre in the refining process.

The function of fibre

Fibre has two main functions in the human digestive tract – filler and mover.

Filler: Fibre provides the structure (both the shape and the texture) of plants. *It is able to absorb from four to six times its own volume of water. Most fruits and vegetables have a high water content and it is the fibre which helps to hold that water and give them their bulk.*

In the digestive tract, fibre takes up

space, creating a soft, spongy mass in the stomach and intestines which gives a feeling of fullness and satisfaction. As *high-fibre foods satisfy the appetite* more quickly, and for longer than low-fibre ones, they protect against overeating and weight problems. One of the most important aids to maintaining a healthy weight is a diet high in unrefined plant foods. This filling function of fibre is one of the most important factors in avoiding obesity and all the problems that go with it, including diabetes, arthritis, heart disease, stroke and cancer.

Mover: Fibre also *stimulates the intestines and this prevents constipation*. Because of its ability to hold water, it keeps the contents of the digestive tract soft, and this enables the muscles of the intestines to move it gently along, without strain or stress. Where fibre is concerned, our intestines are rather like toothpaste tubes – they work smoothly and easily when they are full of soft, moist, bulky material, but they have real difficulties when the contents are dry, hard and small. The insoluble fibre that comes in the outer layers of cereal grains is particularly important as a mover. While low-fibre foods are associated with constipation (food taking three to five days, or even longer, to pass through the system), high-fibre foods pass through far more quickly (24 to 36 hours). This *helps to prevent a long list of constipation-related problems* like haemorrhoids, varicose veins, appendicitis, diverticular disease, and colon cancer. These diseases are very common in Western societies, but almost unheard of in countries where high-fibre diets are the norm.

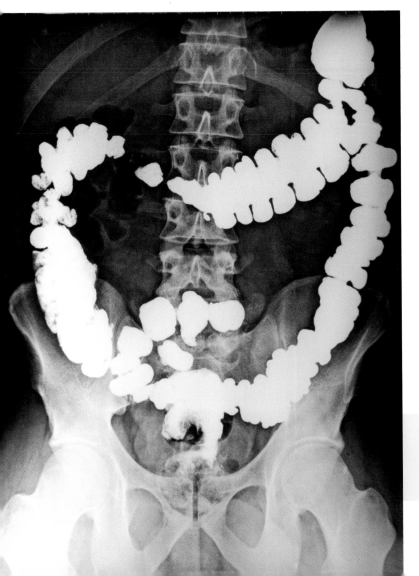

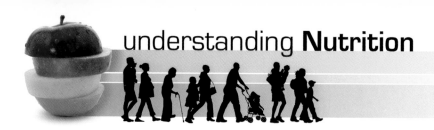
Fibre also serves three other functions:

Blood sugar stabiliser: Fibre slows down the rate at which nutrients are absorbed into the bloodstream, *smoothing out the ups and downs of blood sugar levels.* A stable blood sugar level is important in the relief of hypoglycaemia (low blood sugar), in the control of diabetes (high blood sugar), and, even more importantly, in optimum brain function.

As fibre keeps the intestinal contents moving, there is less chance for it to ferment and produce gases and other unwanted substances, so there is less chance of digestive upsets.

Cholesterol trap: Soluble fibre binds cholesterol and bile acids, which contain cholesterol, in the digestive tract and takes them out of the body. If there is no fibre, they are reabsorbed. This means that *fibre helps to reduce the level of blood cholesterol and thus reduces the risk of heart disease.* Oat bran has been extensively studied in this connection, hence all the packets of oat-rich cereals with health slogans on the supermarket shelves.

Colon protector: Fibre also helps to protect the lining of the colon from harmful food residues. *By speeding things up, fibre reduces the time that cancer-causing substances are in contact with the colon,* and also the time for such substances to be produced.

What foods contain fibre?

All unrefined plant foods contain fibre. Cereal grains are high in fibre, particularly insoluble fibre, so all the whole cereal products, like whole-wheat bread, whole breakfast cereals, whole pasta, brown rice, whole maize meal, barley and rye are rich sources. Fruits are particularly rich in the soluble fibres, but as plant foods contain a

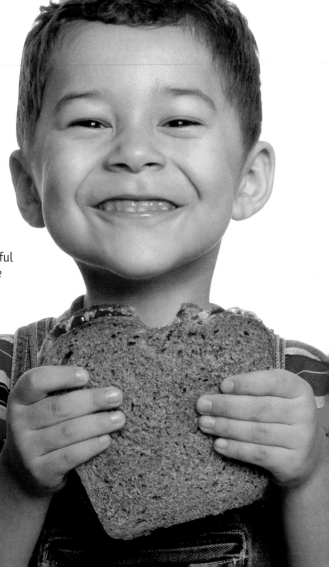

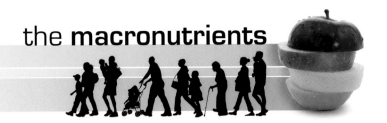

mixture of fibres anyway, there is no need to be concerned about getting the right balance. Beans, lentils and nuts are high in fibre and are quite concentrated foods. Vegetables and fruits have a high water content, so their fibre is less concentrated.

Refined plant foods, like white flour, white sugar and vegetable oils, have lost their fibre. Meat, fish, dairy products and eggs have no fibre. The 'typical' Western diet is composed of around 40% animal products, with most of the remaining part consisting of refined foods. It is therefore very low in fibre, which helps to explain the current epidemic of obesity.

Are fibre supplements necessary?

'With added fibre' (for example bran) is now considered to be a good selling point for refined cereal products. But why remove the fibre to add it back in? The refining processes remove more than fibre anyway: vital minerals and vitamins are also lost.

A diet based on unrefined starches, including a variety of whole grains, fruits, vegetables, and legumes (beans, lentils, and peas), will ensure an abundant supply of fibre. Changing to a more natural diet is a cheaper, safer, and healthier way to go. Focus on whole-grain cereals and breads, fresh fruit and vegetables, with plenty of beans and legumes. This is the easiest and best way to ensure that you get all the fibre you need.

Could one get too much fibre?

Occasionally, a person with a small appetite may not be able to eat enough bulky high-fibre food to supply all the nutrients he needs. This might be the case with the malnourished, the elderly (especially after a lifetime of low-fibre eating) and small children, who would then need to supplement their diet with extra high-calorie, low-fibre foods.

A sudden change from a low-fibre diet to an unrefined plant food diet could certainly give anyone's digestive system a shock, especially if the fluid intake is low. The key is to make changes gradually. The fibre intake can be increased slowly over several weeks. One should always take plenty of fluids, and whenever possible choose a variety of different high-fibre foods.

How much fibre do we need?

There is absolutely no need to make complex calculations. If your diet is based on unrefined starches like bread, potatoes and rice, with generous amounts of vegetables and fruits and small amounts of pulses, nuts and seeds, there will be plenty of fibre.

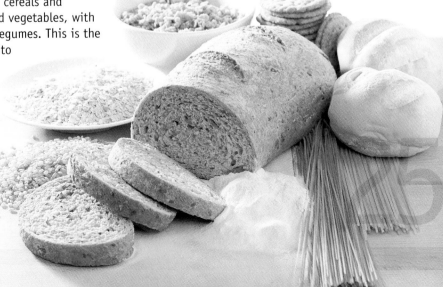

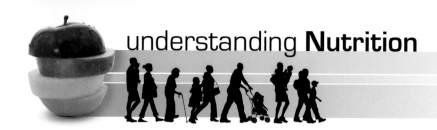

Dennis Burkitt
and the fibre story

Nutritionists and health professionals paid very little attention to fibre until Dennis Burkitt brought it to their attention around 1970. Burkitt was a surgeon whose work in Africa took him to many mission hospitals. He was impressed that the pattern of disease was so different there from what he had been used to at home. In the UK appendicitis was the commonest surgical emergency, but in Africa it was almost unknown. All the commonest conditions in Europe, including varicose veins, piles, gallbladder problems, hiatus hernia and diverticulitis, were rare or unknown. After much work and observation, he concluded that it was diet that made the difference. The African food was simple and unrefined with its full complement of fibre. Observation of the stools produced showed that fibre was the protective factor. So began the fibre revolution in medicine and dietetics.

Protein

Proteins are the building blocks of life, of which we and other living things are made. The word protein, from the Greek word *protos*, meaning 'first', indicates its importance.

Proteins are large and complex molecules, formed from chains of dozens to thousands of amino acids. **All our proteins are made from just twenty amino acids**. Just as there are twenty-six letters in the alphabet, from which an infinite variety of words can be produced, so all the different types of proteins are

produced from these twenty amino acids. These include not only the proteins in the human body, but the proteins in all other living things, including plants.

Amino acids are made of **carbon, hydrogen, oxygen** and **nitrogen**. During digestion, the proteins break down into their component amino acids, which are then transported in the bloodstream to wherever they are needed for growth, repair, maintenance or manufacture. Any surplus to requirements needs to be broken down, as the nitrogen part cannot be stored and must be removed. This gives extra work for the liver, kidneys

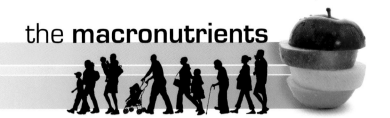

and heart. The remaining part of the amino acid is used either as fuel or converted to fat and stored for later use. When burnt as fuel in the body, one gram of protein produces four calories of energy.

> The **digestive enzymes** that deal with food protein molecules are themselves protein molecules. They act like minuscule scissors, snipping up the food protein molecules into their component amino acids, ready to be absorbed into the blood and carried to where they are needed. There more enzymes enable them to work on growth, repair or manufacture.

> The hormone **insulin** is one of the simplest proteins, containing only forty-eight amino acids. It controls blood sugar levels by acting as a key to unlock the sugar receptor points in the cell walls and letting the sugar in. Without insulin, the sugar does not get into the cells and thus builds up dangerously high levels in the blood – and diabetes develops.

Our bodies contain thousands of different proteins, each with its own individual structure and function. Every cell in our body is built with protein and needs protein for its functions. Proteins are the main components of our muscles, our internal organs, our skin (including our nails and hair). Even our bones are formed in a protein matrix. As well as these structural tissues, proteins have vital roles as hormones and enzymes, enabling our complex biological processes to work, and also as antibodies, combating invaders like bacteria and viruses.

Enzymes are protein molecules that enable specific complex chemical changes to take place quickly and easily in the body. Many are involved in the digestion of food, breaking large molecules down to small components that can be absorbed and transported to where they are needed. **Hormones** act as chemical messengers, travelling throughout the body and controlling the different metabolic activities.

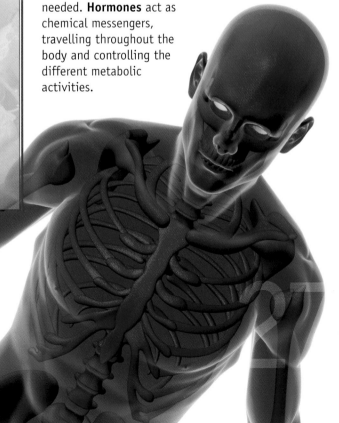

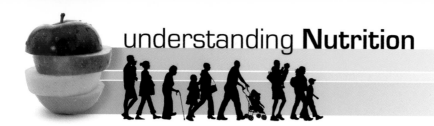

Essential amino acids

For optimum health we need an adequate supply of all the twenty amino acids. The body can manufacture twelve of these. The other eight, the **essential amino acids**, must be supplied in the food.

The animal proteins from meat, fish, poultry, eggs and dairy products, not surprisingly, all contain very similar combinations of amino acids to those found in the human body. The amino acids are in slightly different proportions in plant foods. This led scientists to believe that the animal proteins were better, and that vegetarians were at risk of essential amino acid deficiency. For a while it was thought that some careful food combining was needed to avoid this, but this is now known to be unnecessary. A *variety* of plant proteins from day to day will amply supply all the amino acids needed.

How much protein do we need?

The UK Department of Health recommends 0.8g per kg of body weight a day, so a 70kg man would need 54g and a 60kg woman would need 48g. The World Health Organisation recommends 50g a day as adequate for all adults, including pregnant and nursing mothers. This is a generous allowance and is adequate for growing children too. Our bodies are very efficient at recycling protein so we do not need a large intake, and *it is difficult to go short of protein unless we are actually short of food.*

The real protein problem

For those on a typical Western diet the problems are those associated with protein overdose. The excess protein demands extra work by the liver, to break it down, and by the kidneys to remove urea, the unusable nitrogen residue. This excess workload caused by a regular high-protein intake contributes to problems with the liver, kidneys, and also the heart. A high-protein diet reduces physical endurance. It also takes calcium from the bones, contributing to osteoporosis. While there is evidence that children on high-fat, high-protein diets grow bigger and develop faster, there is also evidence that this accelerated growth is linked to a shorter lifespan.

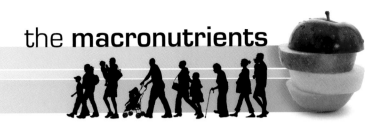

Plant foods are good sources of protein

The most concentrated are pulses – peas, beans and lentils – which are about 30% protein by weight; the grains are next, averaging about 10% protein. As protein is part of the structure of all plant cell walls, all plant foods will contain some. Fruit and vegetables, being high in water and fibre, are low in protein as well as in calories. There are not many calories in broccoli, but 40% of what there are come from protein.

Diets based on an adequate intake of a variety of unrefined starchy foods like grains, rice, potatoes or yams, along with beans and lentils once or twice a day, and generous amounts of vegetables and fruits, will provide plenty of protein, without risk of excess or deficiency. Contrary to what nutritionists thought in the past, completely plant-food diets contain plenty of protein. It is meat eaters whose health is at risk, by getting too much.

Animal foods contain a high proportion of protein, so it is easy to get too much. They also contain more of the sulphur-containing amino acids, which leach calcium out of the bones and contribute to osteoporosis. Animal proteins can transmit animal diseases, and they come with the cholesterol and saturated fat that are associated with degenerative disease. Animal proteins also take longer to digest than plant proteins.

Plant proteins in their natural state come combined with carbohydrate and fibre, so it is less easy to eat too much. They come with healthy fat and without the baggage of cholesterol, saturated fat and other disease-related substances. Plant proteins come with health-promoting phytochemicals, too. *Plant protein is not just as good as animal protein; it is better.*

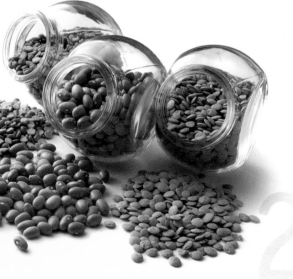

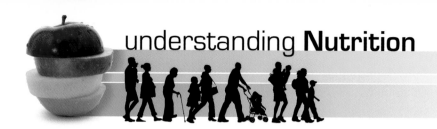

Shall we choose plant or animal protein?

Animal	Plant
Concentrated, no fibre – danger of eating too much	Combined with starch and fibre – more filling, less danger of excess
Comes with cholesterol and saturated fat	No cholesterol and mainly unsaturated fats
High in sulphur-rich amino acids that leach calcium from bones	Low sulphur – bones safe
More vitamins and minerals needed to metabolise it	Brings more vitamins and minerals
Slower digestion, higher acid needed	Easier digestion, less acid needed
No phytochemicals	Phytochemicals that fight ageing and disease
Associated with degenerative diseases and animal borne diseases	Associated with health – plants do not transmit their diseases to humans

Percentage of calories from protein in different foods:

Wheat, oats, rye – average 10%
Legumes – average 30%
Broccoli – 40%
Beef sirloin – 25%
Chicken – 45%
Whole milk – 21%
Skimmed milk – 49%

Environmental and economic factors

Another reason for choosing plant protein is that animal protein is uneconomic to produce.

Cows can turn only 4% of the calories they consume into beef and only 15% into milk. Consider that 7-10lbs of plant protein produce 1lb of animal food and it takes ten times as much land to feed people on animal food as on plant food.

1 acre of land produces 45lbs beef, 270lbs wheat protein, or 400lbs+ soybean protein.

In addition, it takes 100 times more water to produce animal food, mainly to produce the plant foods for the animals to eat. Where land can be used for anything other than grazing, animal food is an expensive use of resources.

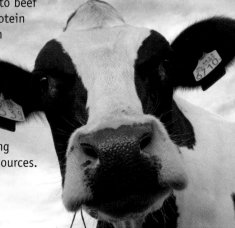

30

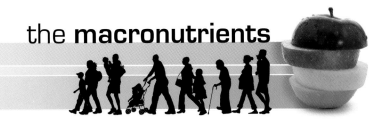

Three protein myths

'Human beings need lots of protein, the more the better' – so said Professor Karl Voigt, the great nineteenth-century pioneer biochemist, who decided that the best way to discover the body's protein requirement was to observe how much protein healthy manual workers chose to eat. This led him to recommend 140g of protein a day for adult males. Only a few years later, Professor Chittenden, in the early 1900s, did a scientific study in which he measured the amount of protein actually used in the body, and he discovered that only 42g a day were needed. His student volunteers tried the low-protein diet with great success, and he himself followed it for the rest of his life. Since that time many other physiologists have confirmed that low-protein diets are adequate, and over the years the recommended daily allowance has gradually dropped. It is now recognised that not only is lower protein *adequate*, but it is *better*, as it is associated with lower incidence of degenerative disease.

'Vegetarians lack protein' – not true. There is plenty of protein in plant foods. The starchy grains and vegetables that form the basis of healthy plant-food diets are high enough in protein to supply most of what is needed. Pulses, nuts and seeds, and even fruit and vegetables, supply the rest. In fact it would need some really careful thought to devise a plant-food diet that was both interesting enough to eat and inadequate in protein. There really isn't any danger if you choose a wide variety of whole foods from day to day, to ensure a good supply of the different amino acids.

'Plant protein is inferior' – this is the old myth about first- and second-class proteins. Animal proteins were considered to be first-class or complete proteins, because the balance of amino acids in them was the most similar to the total balance in our own tissues. Plant proteins are more variable; some have more of one amino acid and less of another than human tissues, so they were designated as second-class or incomplete proteins – and therefore less adequate. The fact is that our cells are able to pick and choose from the pool of amino acids in the bloodstream that results from the digestion of the different types of protein. As long as we eat a *variety* of plant proteins, we are not going to have any problems with a plant-food diet.

31

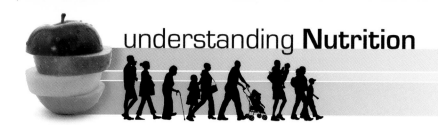

Understanding fats

Fats are a vital part of all living cells, and are essential for maintaining health. However, most people in the rich countries of the West, particularly the UK and the USA, eat much more fat than they need, and the same is true of those who can afford to in the poorer countries of the world. All this fat overloads their systems and causes many serious health problems. The World Health Organisation warns that we now have a global epidemic of obesity – and of all the diseases that go with it.

Functions of fats

Fat provides our main reserve fuel supply. Surplus carbohydrate and protein are both stored in the form of fat. It is the most efficient energy store, providing nine calories of energy per gram. Stored energy from fat keeps us going during long periods of exertion, when food is not available or when the appetite is poor.

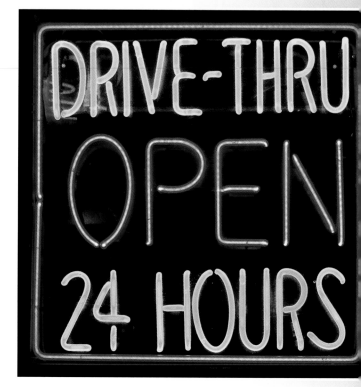

Although excess fat intake and storage seems to be the most serious problem, fat has some essential functions and should not be completely removed from the diet for any length of time.

Very low-fat diets tend to be unappetising, and most people find it very difficult to stay on them.

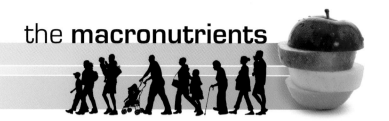

A small amount of fat, especially if provided by natural unrefined plant foods, is important for health.

Fat is necessary as:

☑ Fat keeps us warm: the fat stores under the skin insulate the body from cold.

☑ Fat protects us from injury by providing padding, both under the skin and around the internal organs.

☑ Fat keeps the food in the stomach for a longer time, which helps us to feel satisfied for longer, and so helps to prevent overeating.

☑ Fats enhance the taste, texture and smell of many foods, making them more appetising, and enabling us to maintain healthy diets long term.

☑ Some fats have special functions in the brain and nervous tissues.

☑ Fats are essential to the absorption of the fat-soluble vitamins, A, D, E and K.

Fats belong to the **lipid family** of substances. Most of the fats we eat are **triglycerides** and so is most of the fat stored in our bodies. The other lipids are **phospholipids** and **sterols**. Although we need only small amounts of fats, as they are used in the structure of all our cells, they are essential for growth, maintenance and repair. They also have a role in the manufacture of hormones and related substances which control many aspects of body function, including blood pressure and response to injuries and infections. Cholesterol is one of the sterols.

Nutrition Facts Valeur nutritive		
Per 1/12 pouch (30 g) / Pour 1/12 sac		
Amount / Teneur		% Daily Value / % vale
Calories / Calories 120		
Total Fat / Lipides 2.5 g		
Saturates / satur		
+ Trans / trans		
Polyunsaturate		
Omega-6 / om		
Omega-3 / omé		
Monounsaturates /		
Cholesterol / Cholesté		
Sodium / Sodium 430 m		
Potassium / Potassiur		
Total Carbohydrate /		
Fibre / Fibres 1 g		
Sugars / Sucres 5		
in / Protéine		

Fats are health-promoting when we choose to eat the **right** amount of the **right** kind at the **right** time. Ultra-low-fat diets are not the best. Though they may seem to help middle-aged patients with heart and other problems in the short term, most people find them rather unappetising and difficult to keep up.

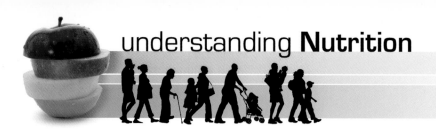

Why is too much fat bad?

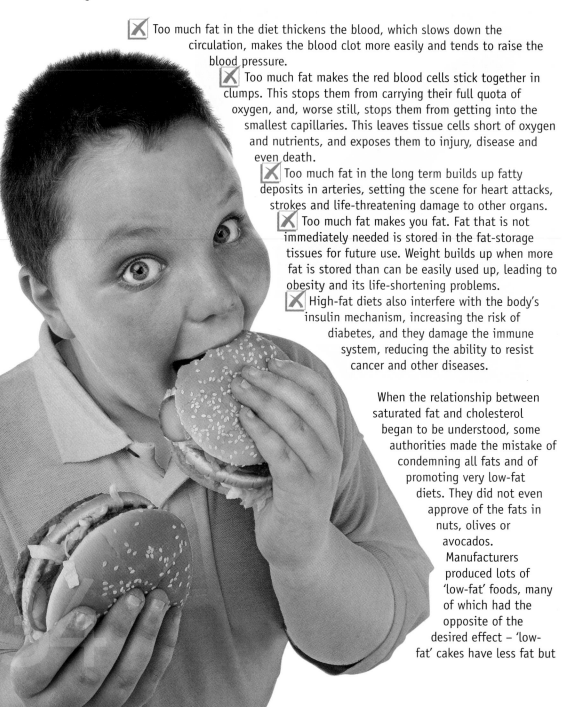

☒ Too much fat in the diet thickens the blood, which slows down the circulation, makes the blood clot more easily and tends to raise the blood pressure.

☒ Too much fat makes the red blood cells stick together in clumps. This stops them from carrying their full quota of oxygen, and, worse still, stops them from getting into the smallest capillaries. This leaves tissue cells short of oxygen and nutrients, and exposes them to injury, disease and even death.

☒ Too much fat in the long term builds up fatty deposits in arteries, setting the scene for heart attacks, strokes and life-threatening damage to other organs.

☒ Too much fat makes you fat. Fat that is not immediately needed is stored in the fat-storage tissues for future use. Weight builds up when more fat is stored than can be easily used up, leading to obesity and its life-shortening problems.

☒ High-fat diets also interfere with the body's insulin mechanism, increasing the risk of diabetes, and they damage the immune system, reducing the ability to resist cancer and other diseases.

When the relationship between saturated fat and cholesterol began to be understood, some authorities made the mistake of condemning all fats and of promoting very low-fat diets. They did not even approve of the fats in nuts, olives or avocados. Manufacturers produced lots of 'low-fat' foods, many of which had the opposite of the desired effect – 'low-fat' cakes have less fat but more sugar and are less satisfying, so more get eaten. Average weights continued to rise, in spite of the low-fat foods.

Gradually, the pieces of the fat puzzle have been fitted together. Happily, we now know that some fat is essential and that we can enjoy eating moderate amounts of plant foods like nuts, seeds, olives and avocados, knowing that they contain important and healthy fats that can actually help to prevent those illnesses that are associated with too much of the wrong sort of fat.

All fats are mixtures of fatty acids. They are described as saturated, monounsaturated or polyunsaturated, according to which type of fatty acid *predominates*.

Saturated fats are solid at room temperature, for example, butter, lard, coconut and palm fat.

Unsaturated fats (mono- and poly-) are oils, liquid at room temperature. Hydrogenation is a process that makes liquid fats solid and more convenient for cooking and spreading.

Biochemistry note

Fats belong to the lipid group of nutrients which come as triglycerides, phospholipids and sterols. Ninety-five percent of the fats in our foods and 99% of the fats in our bodies are triglycerides.

Triglycerides are formed of one glycerol molecule and three fatty acid molecules. They are made from a variety of fatty acids. The mainly saturated ones are solid; the mainly unsaturated ones are liquid.

Fatty acids are chains of carbon atoms with oxygen and hydrogen atoms attached.

Saturated fatty acids have as many hydrogen atoms as possible with no free spaces.

Monounsaturated fatty acids have one free space (a double bond).

Polyunsaturated fatty acids have two free spaces (two double bonds).

The unsaturated fatty acids can be saturated by **hydrogenation**, a process that fits extra hydrogen atoms into the double bonds, changing them from liquid oils to solid fats.

The digestion of fat

Digestion breaks the large fat molecules down to their component parts, which are small enough to be carried in the bloodstream to the places where they are needed. The process begins in the mouth, with enzymes in the saliva. The churning of the stomach helps to mix it in with the rest of the food, but digestion doesn't really get going until the food reaches the small intestine, where bile is added to emulsify the fat – to break down the large fat globules into tiny droplets so the enzymes from the

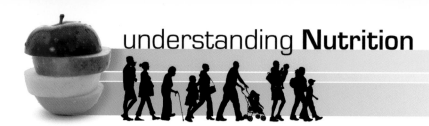

pancreas can start to digest them. When broken down, the small component parts go via the lymph vessels to the bloodstream, which takes them to the destinations where they can be used for energy or any of their other functions. Any excess fat goes to the fat storage cells, where it is rebuilt as triglyceride, and stored until it is needed as fuel. When it is needed, enzymes in the cells break it down and send it out into the bloodstream.

Maintaining healthy levels of cholesterol

As it is part of the structure of all animal cells, all food of animal origin contains cholesterol. The only cholesterol-free animal food is egg white, which does not contain any cell walls. Avoiding animal produce, including flesh foods, dairy and eggs, is the best way to maintain healthy blood cholesterol levels. Saturated fats have a bad reputation because they raise blood cholesterol levels when they are eaten with cholesterol-containing foods. This is a problem, because it is the animal foods that contain the cholesterol and it is mainly the animal foods that contain the saturated fat. Diets have been promoted that try to remove as much saturated fat as possible, but, as long as the animal food is there, the cholesterol problem remains.

Chicken and fish have been advised as healthy alternatives to red meat, because the fat they contain is mainly unsaturated, but of course they still contain cholesterol.

Polyunsaturated fats help to lower cholesterol levels as everyone who reads his margarine or low-fat spread containers knows. But just substituting a high intake of vegetable oils for a high intake of animal fats is not ideal either, because too much fat means too many calories anyway.

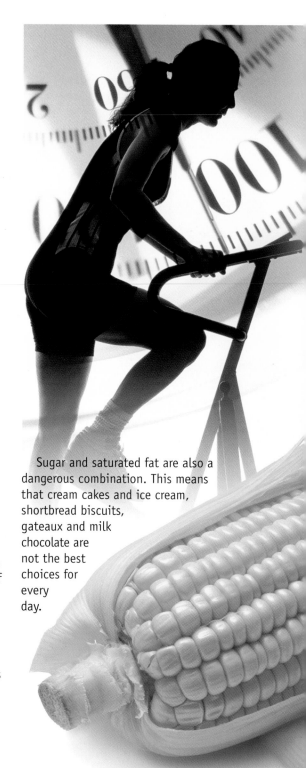

Sugar and saturated fat are also a dangerous combination. This means that cream cakes and ice cream, shortbread biscuits, gateaux and milk chocolate are not the best choices for every day.

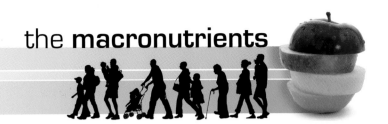

Whole plant foods, prepared in as simple and natural a way as possible, are the answer to lowering cholesterol safely. They do not contain any cholesterol at all and they contain fibre that helps to trap cholesterol and move it out of the body.

Food is not the whole story so far as lowering cholesterol is concerned, however. Exercise, sunlight, stress control, the avoidance of poisons such as alcohol, tobacco and caffeine, all have vital roles to play in keeping the blood cholesterol at healthy levels.

Which are the best fats to eat?

Fats as they come in whole plant foods are best. Refining concentrates them to levels where it is almost impossible not to over-consume them. Take sweet corn, for example. It takes twelve or more corncobs to produce a tablespoonful of corn oil. No one would want to eat twelve corncobs, but it would be very easy to add their equivalent in a couple of tablespoonfuls of mayonnaise, which is mainly oil, to a meal and hardly notice it. Nuts, seeds, olives and avocados are delicious examples of natural high-fat plant foods, which, in moderation, can be a healthy part of a plant-food diet.

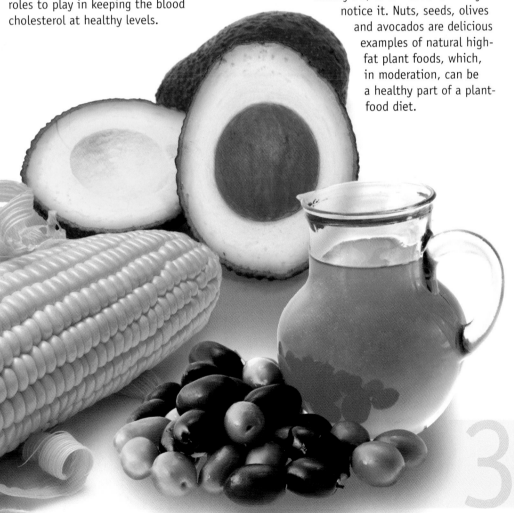

37

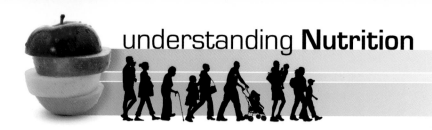

Essential fatty acids

These are **linoleic (omega 6) acid** and **linolenic (omega 3) acid**. It is essential to get them from food because the body cannot make them. They are very important in maintaining both mental and physical health. Their functions include:

▶ Control of **factors relating to heart disease and stroke,** such as blood pressure, blood clotting and blood levels of fats, including cholesterol.

▶ Maintaining the **immune system** and its functions in healing and in preventing allergies, infections and cancer.

▶ Development and maintenance of the **brain and nervous system,** including memory, intelligence and mental health.

There are plenty of these essential fatty acids in a variety of plant foods, particularly in the oils of nuts and seeds, grains and green, leafy vegetables. Vegetable cooking oils are particularly high in the omega 6 fats. Flaxseed, walnuts, pumpkinseed and rapeseed are high in omega 3. Fish is also high in omega 3.

Our bodies need five or six times as much of the omega 6 as the omega 3. This is the sort of ratio in which they occur in whole plant foods. Problems arise because when foods are refined, the ratio changes. Ordinary vegetable cooking oils are very rich in omega 6, and the typical Western diet, with its high use of vegetable oils and low use of whole nuts and seeds, provides far more omega 6 than is needed.

To re-balance this we are advised to eat more oily fish, but unfortunately they are very prone to the effects of pollution. **The best solution is to limit the use of refined oils and choose a whole plant food diet, including plenty of unrefined cereals, nuts, seeds and green, leafy vegetables.**

Biochemistry note

The essential omega 6 and omega 3 fatty acids are polyunsaturated, and the numbers 3 and 6 refer to the fact that the spaces or double bonds in the unsaturated fatty-acid molecules are at the third or sixth carbon atom. These fats are the ones with special functions in the heart, circulation and brain. The essential linoleic and linolenic acids both belong to this group. The ideal proportion of omega 6 to omega 3 is 5:1 or 6:1. A typical Western diet provides far more omega 6 than is needed, most of it from refined vegetable oils. Solution: avoid refined vegetable oils and eat whole, natural, plant foods.

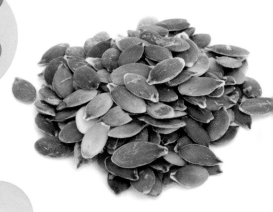

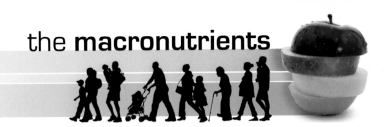

What about omega supplements?

Commercial omega 3 supplements are not necessary to correct the balance of omega 6 and omega 3. To reduce the proportion of omega 6, simply cut out (or reduce drastically) the refined cooking oils. To increase the proportion of omega 3, supplement your diet not with pills but with omega 3-rich foods. The richest source of omega 3 is flaxseed; the next is walnuts. Soya, pumpkinseeds and green, leafy vegetables are also sources. A simple way to include them in your diet is to sprinkle walnuts, pumpkinseeds and ground flaxseed on breakfast cereals.

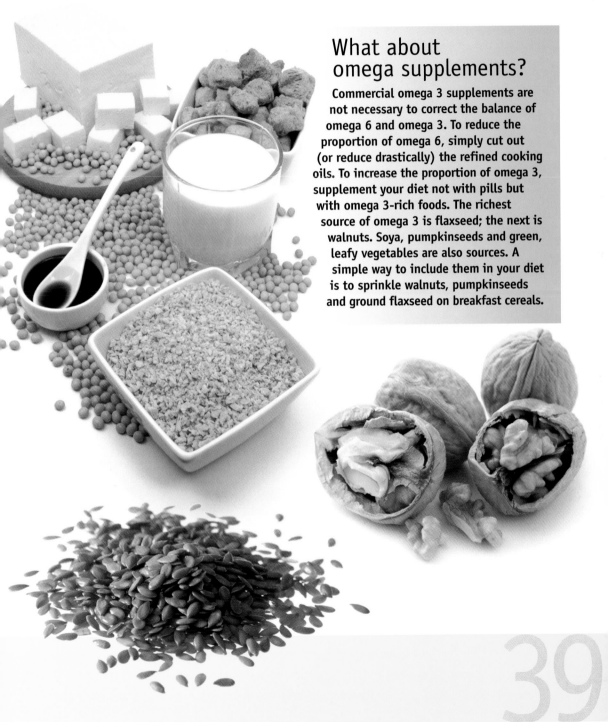

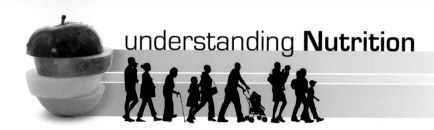

Hydrogenated fats and trans fats

Oils can be turned into solid fats by hydrogenation, a process where the oils are heated to a high temperature in the presence of hydrogen. Hydrogen atoms are added to the fat molecules at the double bonds, turning the liquid unsaturated fats into solid saturated fats. The solid fats are more convenient for spreading and cooking, but they now have all the disadvantages of saturated fats – they raise cholesterol levels and are associated with an increased risk of heart disease. The process also produces trans fats, which are even more worrying.

Some of the fat molecules do not get hydrogenised, but get twisted into a different shape: these are the trans fats. The body cannot use them in the normal way, and they are associated with higher levels of heart disease and possibly with cancer. Authorities view trans fats as unnecessary and unnatural, and food manufacturers vie with one another to prove that their products are the most trans fat free.

How to avoid trans fats

Although most margarine is now free from trans fats and is labelled accordingly, trans-fat-rich shortening is still widely used in baking: this means beware of bought cakes, pies and biscuits, and read the labels carefully if you are buying solid fats for home baking. The best plan is to avoid refined and processed fats as far as possible, choosing unrefined plant foods as the basis of your diet.

What about frying?

The high temperatures needed to fry food have an effect on the oils used. Most of the commonly used vegetable oils are unstable at high temperatures. This means that their chemistry alters and free radicals, trans fats and other harmful substances form. At the same time, antioxidants and other healthy elements are destroyed. Every time the oil is re-used, more damage is done, and these changes are associated with damage to the immune system, contributing to cancer and other degenerative diseases. Deep-fat frying is not recommended, and if it must be done the oil should be used only once.

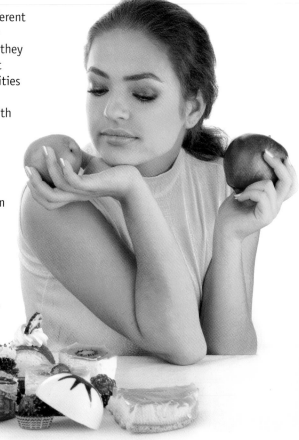

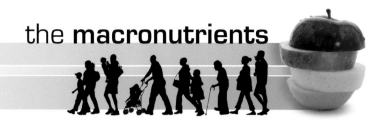
How much fat can we safely eat?

It is much less complicated than it seems. The experts at the WHO advise that we get not less than 15% and not more that 35% of our calories from fat. The average Western diet varies between 35 and 45% of calories from fats. A varied diet of mainly whole, unrefined plant foods solves the problem. There is no need to worry about calories or percentages if you choose the right food. Choosing a good variety of different unrefined plant foods each day, including some of the high-fat ones, provides around 15 to 20% of calories from fat, well within the safe limits for most people.

Which fats should we eat in addition to the natural oils as they come in whole plant foods?

Olive oil, a monounsaturated fat, is associated with lower cholesterol levels and most people can safely use it in moderation. Olive oil differs in several ways from other vegetable fats and oils. Virgin olive oil is not refined but simply pressed out of the olives. It is much more stable at high temperatures, avoiding the trans fat problem. It also contains its own valuable health promoting phytochemicals. The best sort is the cold-pressed extra virgin oil, which is not refined or processed, and contains more of the phytochemicals than the cheaper processed olive oils.

Sunflower, soy, rapeseed and the other commonly used vegetable oils are highly refined, a process involving very high temperatures with the danger of trans fat formation.

The cold-pressed varieties are usually hard to find, and expensive. The solution is to use as little refined oil as possible. Active children and young people need not be as careful as adults, but those who are overweight or are already suffering from heart or other degenerative disease would be best to avoid it altogether.

N.B. Olive oil is a concentrated food, but not a refined one. It's usually a lot more expensive than other oils, but that should not be a problem if we use only a small amount of it. Should people with heart and arterial disease use olive oil? Some authorities would say no oil at all for this group, but others would say, by all means use it (sparingly if they need to lose weight) because it is an important part of the heart-protecting Mediterranean diet.

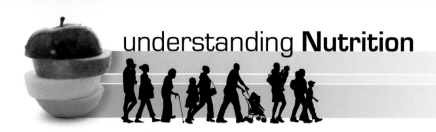

The Mediterranean diet

People from the south of Italy, Greece and other Mediterranean areas suffer less from heart disease than people from Northern Europe. This has been attributed to their diet with its olive oil, fresh fruit and vegetables and red wine. Olive oil, fruit and vegetables are certainly associated with healthier hearts, and the red wine provides resveratrol, a red phytochemical found in red grape skins, and present in fresh grapes and unfermented grape juice as well as wine. They also eat more fish, and less red meat and dairy produce. And, of course, the extra sunshine and fresh air could have something to do with it.

More about cholesterol

In recent years cholesterol has acquired a bad reputation, despite its essential role in our bodies. The average human body contains about 150mg of cholesterol, 7% of which is in the bloodstream. Our bodies are designed to produce all the cholesterol they need and to cope with some extra from the diet. It's only when there is too much cholesterol that problems arise, which happens when we take in more than our bodies can deal with. Almost everyone knows about the link between high blood cholesterol levels and heart disease, but not so many know about the good things that cholesterol does. The cholesterol in the bloodstream is on its way to perform many important tasks.

What is cholesterol for?

It forms part of the structure of cell walls where it helps to regulate the passage of substances in and out. Cholesterol is also a raw material for the manufacture of vitamin D (essential for strong bones and many other health-maintenance functions) and adrenal, pituitary and reproductive hormones. It is also present in bile which enables us to digest fats and absorb fat-soluble vitamins. Another role is in tissue repair. These are just some of the vitally important functions of cholesterol, but because of its role in heart disease, most people think it is something very bad, and are unaware that it is essential to life.

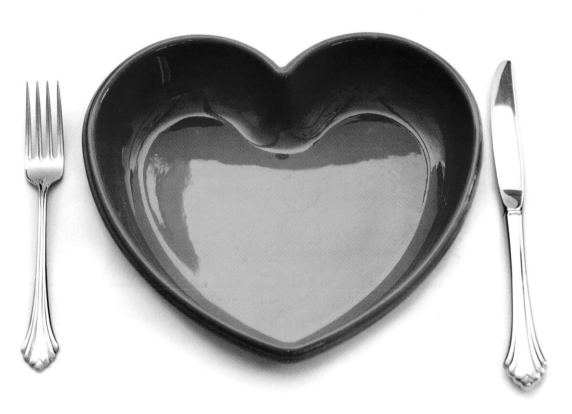

Good and bad cholesterol

Cholesterol in our bodies comes in several forms and the main ones are HDL and LDL (high and low density lipoprotein). The LDL transports cholesterol towards the tissues, including the arteries, and high levels are associated with higher levels of heart disease and stroke. HDL transports cholesterol to the liver for breakdown and removal. High levels of HDL are associated with less heart disease and stroke. Both sorts of cholesterol are necessary for health, and trouble comes when there is too much or when the balance is wrong.

Which foods contain cholesterol?

As it is present in all animal cells, it is present in all animal produce, with the sole exception of egg white. Plants do not manufacture it, so **there is no cholesterol in any plant food.**

How much cholesterol is it safe to eat?

It depends on the individual. Some people can eat a lot of animal produce and still stay well; others would be better to eat none at all. Most people who eat the typical, refined, high-fat, animal-food-rich Western diet eat a great deal of cholesterol, raising the amount in their blood to potentially dangerous levels.

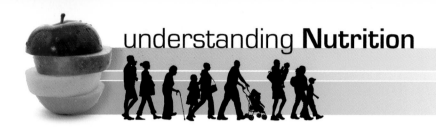

What is a safe blood cholesterol level?

This is a case where taking the national average is not a good guide. In the UK the average level is above the recommended safe level of 5.2 or less.

Saturated versus unsaturated fats

Cholesterol is more dangerous in the presence of saturated fat, which is the main kind of fat in red meat, dairy produce and eggs. Fish and poultry are considered to be more healthy because they have more of the unsaturated fats, but they still contain cholesterol. Awareness of the health risks associated with saturated fats has given rise to a whole industry, devoted to producing margarines from polyunsaturated fats. These oils, like corn and sunflower, can help to reduce blood cholesterol levels, but it's not all good news, as a higher intake of polyunsaturated fats, though associated with less heart disease, is also associated with an increase in liver disorders and cancer.

Do saturated plant fats raise cholesterol?

Coconut and palm oil are saturated fats and they can increase blood cholesterol levels if they are part of a diet containing cholesterol, so meat eaters and ovo-lacto vegetarians should be careful. Those on a completely plant-food diet do not eat cholesterol, so they should not normally need to worry about small amounts of these foods.

How does cholesterol damage the heart?

The first step is damage to the lining of the coronary arteries. One of the functions of cholesterol is to help with tissue healing, and it forms 'patches' that cover up the damage until healing takes place. If the damaging conditions persist, more of these 'patches' are applied, one on top of another, until eventually, after many years, the arteries become narrow and obstructed, and the scene is set for a heart attack. When the same thing happens to arteries supplying the brain, the scene is set for a stroke. But what causes the original damage? One theory is that lack of vitamin C starts the process, and that high blood levels of cholesterol simply compound it. We now know that heart attacks happen when there is some sort of inflammation present as well as the narrowed arteries.

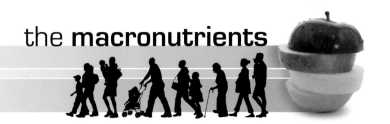

Can diet lower the blood cholesterol level?

Cholesterol levels *can* be lowered by our eating less meat and dairy produce and fewer eggs and refined foods. The best option is an unrefined plant-food diet. Because plant foods are high in fibre (which binds cholesterol and removes it from the body), low in saturated fat and cholesterol-free, increasing the quantity of fruits, nuts, grains (especially oats) and vegetables (particularly beans) makes a good start. It's best to avoid the use of free fats (refined oils, margarine and so on) where possible. Olive oil, which is mainly a monounsaturated fat, is the healthiest fat, and even has cholesterol-lowering properties itself.

A total health programme to control cholesterol

Although cholesterol-lowering drugs are now frequently used, the ideal way to lower cholesterol is a healthy, unrefined plant-food diet which is part of a total health programme that includes regular exercise, lots of water to drink, abstinence from harmful substances – and a sense of humour!

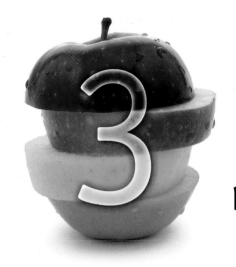

3

The micronutrients

The vitamins

One dictionary definition is 'organic substances of which minute quantities are essential for the proper functioning of the body, and which must be supplied in the diet'. They are powerful substances with specific functions, whose absence causes serious and even life-threatening problems, ranging from blindness (vitamin A lack), scurvy (vitamin C lack) and the deformed bones of rickets (vitamin D lack) to spina bifida, the birth defect due to deficiency of folate, (one of the B group of vitamins).

Vitamins do not provide energy themselves. They act as helpers in metabolic processes, and are involved in almost every action of the body.

Vitamins were discovered when scientists found that certain, once common diseases could be cured by mysterious dietary factors. Gradually, in the early years of the twentieth century, they discovered this group of varied substances that are needed to maintain life and health and to prevent disease.

The word vitamin means 'vital amine'

vita = (necessary for) life
amine = nitrogen-containing compound

Scientists thought all of the new substances would be amines, and, although they are not, the collective name stuck.

46

the micronutrients

Vitamins come as individual units. Unlike carbohydrates, fats and proteins, they do not need to be broken down in the digestive system, but are ready for use, or are easily activated. They come in tiny amounts which are measured not in grams but in milligrams and micrograms.

They all have their own specific roles in growth and maintenance of all parts of the body. Deficiencies cause dire problems that are relieved dramatically when the deficiency is corrected. Although each has its own work,

the vitamins work as a team, and also interact with minerals like calcium, selenium, phosphorus and zinc.

It is important to choose vitamin-rich food, but how much the body can take in and use also depends on how efficiently the digestive system absorbs them, how much is already in the body and what other foods are eaten at the same time. Because some of the vitamins are delicate and easily destroyed by air, heat and light, how the foods are stored and prepared is also important.

Preventing vitamin loss

As vitamins are sensitive to heat, light and air, so the content of a given food can be affected by its freshness, and both the length of time and the temperature at which it is stored. Fresh foods are best when eaten as soon as possible after picking. If they cannot be eaten soon, they need to be stored in a cool, dark place. Vitamins in cut surfaces of foods are oxidised on exposure to air, so cut fruits and vegetables should be covered and stored in airtight containers. Such foods should be prepared as short a time before eating as possible.

Heat destroys vitamins, and water dissolves them, so fresh foods should be cooked as quickly as possible, in as little water as possible, and that water should be saved and used. Quick steaming, stir cooking and baking ensure minimal vitamin loss. Many vegetables are easier to digest when cooked, and when carefully stored and cooked, they still contain most of their vitamins, so it is not necessary to eat everything raw. Grains are different: they need long, slow cooking to break down the cells and release the vitamins.

Vitamins come as two types: water-soluble and fat-soluble.

The water-soluble vitamins are the **vitamin B group** and **vitamin C**. They circulate freely in the body fluids, and the kidneys easily remove any surplus in the urine, so unless excessive doses of supplements are taken, there is no danger of toxicity. On the other hand, because they are not stored in the body, a constant supply is needed and should be eaten most days.

The fat-soluble vitamins are **A, D, E** and **K.** They come in animal produce as well as with the fats in plants, and are absorbed along with fats and oils. Once in the body, they go to storage areas like the liver and fat-storage tissues, to be released when needed. Because our bodies can store them, we do not need to eat them so often. As they are not soluble in water, they are much less easy to get rid of, and, as any excess tends to be stored, the unwise use of supplements can cause toxicity.

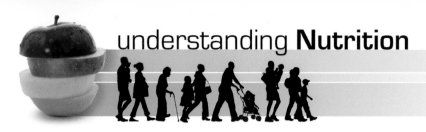

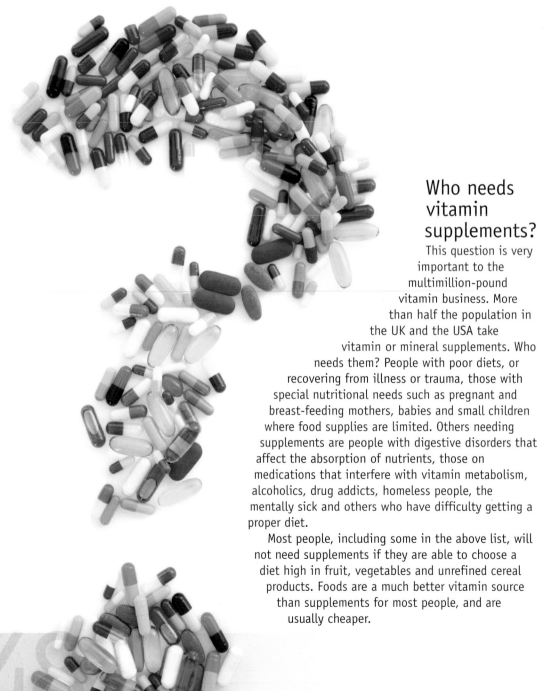

Who needs vitamin supplements?

This question is very important to the multimillion-pound vitamin business. More than half the population in the UK and the USA take vitamin or mineral supplements. Who needs them? People with poor diets, or recovering from illness or trauma, those with special nutritional needs such as pregnant and breast-feeding mothers, babies and small children where food supplies are limited. Others needing supplements are people with digestive disorders that affect the absorption of nutrients, those on medications that interfere with vitamin metabolism, alcoholics, drug addicts, homeless people, the mentally sick and others who have difficulty getting a proper diet.

Most people, including some in the above list, will not need supplements if they are able to choose a diet high in fruit, vegetables and unrefined cereal products. Foods are a much better vitamin source than supplements for most people, and are usually cheaper.

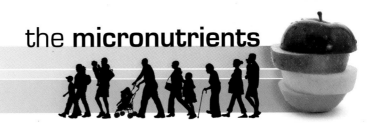

The water-soluble vitamins

Vitamin B complex

The B vitamin group work as coenzymes, facilitating the work of enzymes in every cell in the body. They are active in carbohydrate, fat and protein metabolism, and in making the DNA for new cells.

The B vitamins work in co-operation. They help in the metabolism of energy production. The different members of the group work with different enzymes in the many stages of the processes that release energy from the fuel foods. This means that they are involved in the metabolism of all our trillions of cells, and their deficiencies cause a wide range of problems. Because they are widely distributed in many kinds of food, and have such a wide range of functions, apart from B12, *individual* deficiencies are rare nowadays, unless diets are very restricted. On the other hand, *general* B complex deficiencies are not rare, and could account for many vague symptoms of poor health, including lack of energy, unexplained aches and pains, irritability, and so on.

The group members are **thiamine (B1), riboflavin (B2), niacin (B3), biotin, pantothenic acid, B6 whose best-known component is pyridoxine, folate (folic acid), and vitamin B12.**

Thiamine was discovered in 1926. It was the missing factor in beriberi, a disease with weakness and paralysis, that is still occasionally found in alcoholics and other severely malnourished people. In 1926 it was very common in Southeast Asia where many people had little other than white rice to eat. The process of polishing the rice removed the nutritious bran with the thiamine that was needed to prevent the problem.

Niacin is particularly involved with energy metabolism in the skin, digestive tract and nervous system. Deficiency caused the now rare disease pellagra, characterised by diarrhoea, dermatitis, and, if not treated, dementia and death.

Pantothenic acid is impressive in that it is involved in at least a hundred different steps in the production of lipids, neurotransmitters and steroids.

Pyridoxine (B6) has a vital role in the activity of many enzymes, and as well as energy production it's involved in red blood cell formation and the nervous system. It converts the amino acid tryptophan to the neurotransmitter serotonin, which is important for healthy nerves and brain. Deficiency symptoms include weakness, irritability and insomnia. Megavitamin therapies sometimes recommend doses of many times the recommended daily intake and these can cause toxicity, with damage to nerves in the legs and feet.

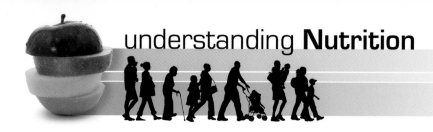

B12 and folate are closely related.
Vitamin B12 is needed to convert the folate to its active form. **Folate** has special functions in the synthesis of DNA for new cells, including red blood cells. Folate also helps to prevent heart disease, but it is best known for helping to prevent the birth defect spina bifida, where the baby's spine is not properly formed, leaving the spinal cord exposed to damage. Deficiency can also cause anaemia with large red cells, weakness, digestive disorders and other problems.

B12 works as a coenzyme in new-cell production and nerve cell maintenance. It also is necessary for forming red blood cells, and it has its own special role in the nervous system, protecting nerve-fibre sheaths. Deficiency of B12 can produce a variety of problems, including anaemia, and, if not corrected, can cause irreversible damage to peripheral nerves. Another complication is that a good supply of folate can mask a B12 deficiency by keeping the blood normal, but letting the nerve damage progress. Pernicious anaemia is a disease where B12 cannot be absorbed; fatal before the discovery of B12, but it is now very easily treated with regular injections.

Apart from B12, **all the B vitamins are widely distributed in small amounts in frequently eaten plant foods, particularly unrefined cereals,** and in some animal produce. Folate is found in green leafy vegetables, legumes and seeds, and, for meat eaters, in liver.

B12 is different and there is rather a mystery about it and considerable controversy. It is not made by either plants or animals, but by bacteria. All animal produce, being rich in bacteria, contains B12. Plant foods usually contain none at all. This raises a very interesting question as to where healthy lifelong vegans get their B12 from if they do not get it from their food. As bacteria are almost everywhere except on plant foods, could they get it as a 'contaminant', as even clean tap water can contain it? Or could it be produced by bacteria inside their bodies, on their teeth, or in their digestive tracts? Much speculation surrounds this topic. Blood levels of B12 tend to be lower in vegans and vegetarians than in meat eaters, but this could be because these lower levels reflect a lower need, or even a healthier level, as long-term vegans tend to be healthy, energetic people. Most of this research has been done in the West, where food supplies now tend to be super hygienic, and even friendly bacteria are excluded from the irradiated, washed and plastic-wrapped produce on the supermarket shelves.

Deficiencies of B12 are more often due to poor absorption than to inadequate intake; they are not at all rare, even in meat eaters whose intake is high. The problem is that deficiencies develop very gradually, with a range of possible early symptoms such as weakness, tiredness, irritability and vague numbness and tingling in the feet and legs, which can be overlooked.

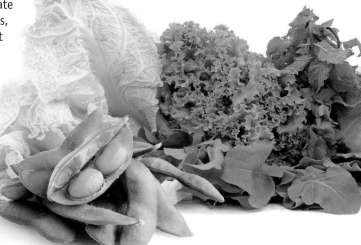

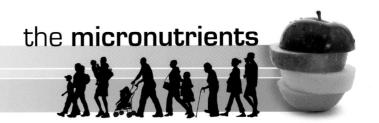

Unfortunately, the nerve damage can be permanent if it's not recognised and corrected in time.

To prevent such disasters, B12 is added to some foods such as yeast extract, soya milk and even cornflakes. Some recommend that all vegans and strict vegetarians of whatever age take regular supplements, the recommended dosage ranging from 4-10 micrograms daily, depending on to which authority you listen. Both are minute amounts; very little is needed because the body recycles and stores it very efficiently, an average person having enough for several years stored in his liver. The UK Vegan Society have done extensive research into this topic, and they recommend that vegans get at least 3mcg a day from B12 fortified foods or take a daily supplement of 10mcg, or, because B12 is absorbed much less efficiently in larger amounts, a weekly supplement of 2000mcg. Blood tests for B12 are rather unreliable, so they recommend that any strict vegans not taking a supplement should have an annual methyl malonic urine test* to ensure that they are not deficient.

NOTE
* Methyl malonic urine tests are available from **Biolab, The Stone House, London, W1W 6DB.**

Strict vegetarians and vitamin B12

Vegans do occasionally have problems with absorbing enough B12 and all who start on a long-term, totally plant-food diet should be aware of this and get their B12 blood levels checked each year until they are sure they have stabilised. **It's especially important for vegan pregnant mothers and their babies to have this test, because there are occasionally cases of B12 deficient mothers having seriously ill B12 deficient babies.**

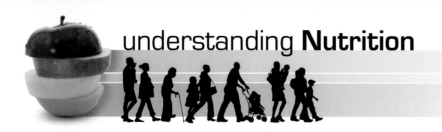
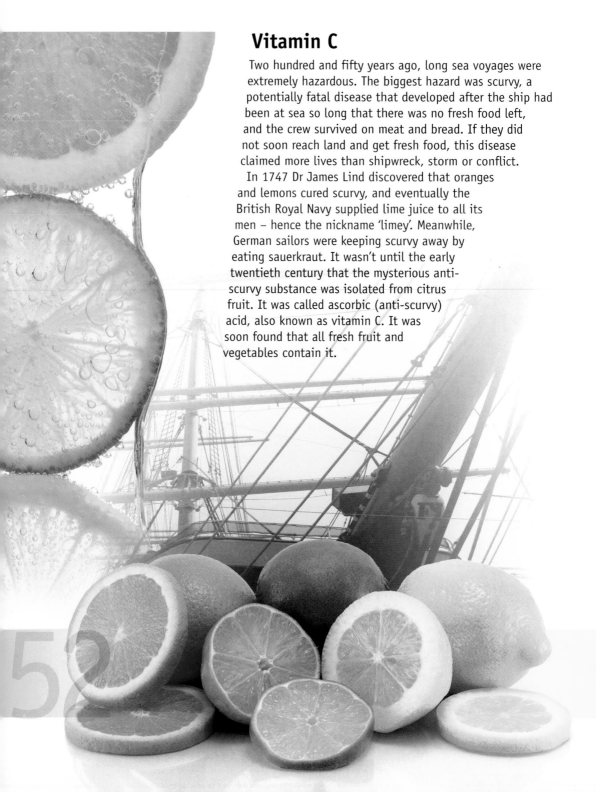

Vitamin C

Two hundred and fifty years ago, long sea voyages were extremely hazardous. The biggest hazard was scurvy, a potentially fatal disease that developed after the ship had been at sea so long that there was no fresh food left, and the crew survived on meat and bread. If they did not soon reach land and get fresh food, this disease claimed more lives than shipwreck, storm or conflict.

In 1747 Dr James Lind discovered that oranges and lemons cured scurvy, and eventually the British Royal Navy supplied lime juice to all its men – hence the nickname 'limey'. Meanwhile, German sailors were keeping scurvy away by eating sauerkraut. It wasn't until the early twentieth century that the mysterious anti-scurvy substance was isolated from citrus fruit. It was called ascorbic (anti-scurvy) acid, also known as vitamin C. It was soon found that all fresh fruit and vegetables contain it.

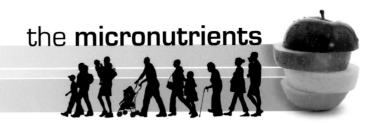

The role of vitamin C

It is important for the **circulation**, as it helps maintain the blood vessels, and helps with the absorption of iron and the formation of haemoglobin (the red oxygen-carrying pigment in the blood). It's also important for the **skin**, and for **every organ** in the body, because it helps to form and maintain **collagen** – the fibrous protein which is the basis of all the connective and structural tissues. It helps with **fighting infection** and with **wound healing.** In addition, it is **a powerful antioxidant, helping to prevent ageing, heart disease and cancer.**

Excess is possible because of megavitamin therapy. Some therapies recommend up to 12g of vitamin C a day. Such large amounts can over-acidify the urine and cause kidney stones to form.

As a water-soluble vitamin it is damaged by air, heat and water, so cooking and storage methods are important.

Food sources of vitamin C

Fresh fruit and vegetables are the most important sources. Dried fruits and vegetables have lost most of their vitamin C. Frozen fruit and vegetables retain most of it.

Even tinned fruit and bottled fruit juices retain some, though often extra is added. Cereals, pulses, nuts, dairy produce and meats have little or no natural vitamin C.

Recommended daily intake

An intake of 10mg of vitamin C to avoid scurvy, 30mg to run normal metabolism. Smokers need more than non-smokers, and so do those who are ill or recovering from illness. At 100g a day, in normal people, including smokers, all tissues are saturated with vitamin C and any excess is excreted. A whole-plant-food diet, with plenty of fruits and vegetables, some of them raw, will ensure an abundant supply of vitamin C.

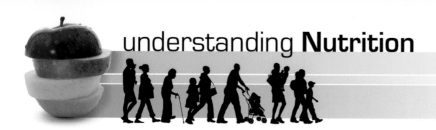
The fat-soluble vitamins

These come with the fats and oils in foods. As they are insoluble in water, they need bile for absorption, and they are transported in the body by protein-carrying molecules. Any excess is stored in the liver or fat storage tissues, ready for future use. This means that a fresh supply is not needed as often as with the water-soluble vitamins, but it does also mean that they are not so easy to get rid of. Toxicity is possible, so supplements should be used with care.

Vitamin A and beta-carotene

Vitamin A occurs only in animals. Plant foods contain beta-carotene, the vitamin A precursor, which, when eaten, is converted to vitamin A. Beta carotene is a bright-orange pigment, first isolated from carrots, hence its name. **Beta-carotene is converted to vitamin A as it is needed. Any that is not converted to vitamin A is used as a powerful antioxidant.**

Vitamin A roles

This vitamin works like a hormone, promoting protein synthesis and cell development, which is particularly important in maintaining the **skin**, the **linings and coverings of organs, reproduction, growth** and **vision**. It has two vital roles in the eye: first keeping the cornea crystal clear, and, second, promoting the transmission of the visual image from the retina to the brain.

54

Vitamin A deficiencies are common in developing countries where malnutrition is rife, and give rise to specific problems, particularly in children. It is the commonest cause of blindness in children, and the World Health Organisation has highlighted a specific problem with measles, as Vitamin A deficient children suffer more severely with this disease. Vitamin A deficiency is possible in the developed world too. Fast foods contain very little. Those on an exclusively junk food diet can expect eye problems, starting with night blindness – not being able to see in the dark – and problems with bones, teeth, eyes, and poor resistance to infections.

Vitamin A toxicity is possible if supplements are used excessively. Beta-carotene does not have this problem, because any surplus is simply stored in the skin, and not converted to vitamin A. People who are supplementing their diet with massive quantities of carrot juice could have a problem, however – their skin could turn orange, but fortunately only temporarily.

Sources of vitamin A – animal produce.

Sources of beta-carotene – plant foods. This bright orange pigment is very widely distributed in plants, and is especially rich in orange-coloured foods like carrots, cantaloupe melons, sweet potatoes, apricots, and also in dark vegetables and fruits, such as green, leafy vegetables and blue and black berries, where the orange colour is masked by the other pigments.

Vitamin D

This vitamin is different from other vitamins in that it is formed in the skin in sunlight, so those who get enough sunlight make their own and do not need to get it from food.

The vitamin D precursor is made from cholesterol, and when the skin is exposed to sunlight it changes to the active vitamin. Skin colour is important, because the skin pigment melanin screens out the sun's rays. Fair-skinned people need an average of ten minutes' sunlight on the hands and face each day to provide adequate vitamin D. Dark skins need more exposure, perhaps fifteen to twenty minutes a day. This is easy for people in sunny climates, but more difficult in cloudy northern countries like the UK, where the winter sunshine is not strong enough for vitamin D production, especially in dark-skinned people. Ideally, with plenty of time outdoors in the summer, a person will have enough vitamin D stored to last the winter; however, as people age their bodies are less efficient, and as vitamin D doesn't occur in plant foods, some people, especially if they spend a lot of their time indoors, may need a supplement in the winter.

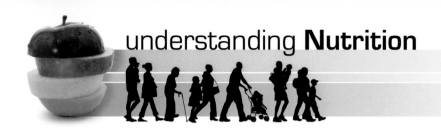

The role of vitamin D

Vitamin D is a member of a large group of nutrients, including vitamins A, C and K which, along with hormones and the minerals calcium and phosphorus, work together to build and maintain bone.

Vitamin D increases the absorption of calcium and phosphorus from the digestive tract and makes it available to the bones. It is now known to have numerous other health promoting and disease preventing functions, many of which have only recently been recognised.

Scientists are discovering that Vitamin D has a much wider range of action than they had thought. As well as its action on bones, it has important effects on the immune system, the heart and circulation and even the brain. Its deficiency is now thought to contribute to many degenerative diseases, including heart disease and cancer. As well as helping to prevent these, vitamin D has been shown to protect the skin against sunburn, and the brain and nervous system against Parkinson's disease, multiple sclerosis, stroke and even memory loss. It also strengthens the immune system to resist both chronic autoimmune disease and everyday infections like coughs, colds and flu.

Vitamin D deficiency has long been known to interfere with bone growth, causing children to develop rickets, a condition where their bones are soft and weak. Adults can develop osteomalacia where their bones become soft and weak, too. However, recent research indicates that vitamin D has a far wider influence and its deficiency is now thought to be involved with many degenerative and other conditions.

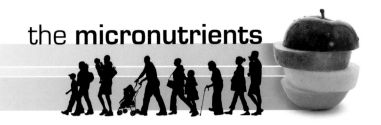

Food sources of vitamin D

The natural sources are all animal ones – dairy produce, meat, eggs, liver and oily fish. Fish oils are the richest source.
Unfortunately, fish in polluted waters store heavy metals in their livers, so fish liver oil is no longer an ideal choice. Vitamin D is added to some foods, particularly margarines.

Who needs supplements?

Some people, especially the elderly, who live in cool, cloudy northern countries and spend most of their time indoors may need to take a supplement to see them through the winter months.

Toxicity is possible with excess intake from supplements and can cause very serious problems. Excess vitamin D is stored in the body and can cause calcium to be mobilised from bones and deposited in unsuitable areas, such as major arteries where it can cause fatal problems, including kidney failure.

How dangerous is sunlight?

Sunlight is necessary for the production of vitamin D in the skin, and sunscreens above factor 8 prevent vitamin D synthesis. But sunshine is also linked with skin ageing and, worse still, skin cancer, and light-skinned people are advised to use sunscreens generously. So what are they to do? The problem is not sunlight, but *excess* sunlight. Sun*burn* is not only painful and unsightly, but it can set the scene for skin cancer to develop many years later. A healthy sun*tan* protects the skin from burning. And there is another factor: whole unrefined plant foods contain phytochemicals that help to prevent all kinds of damage, whereas the high-sugar, high-fat, high-animal-protein Western diet, along with smoking, alcohol and other immune-system depressants, has the opposite effect. To avoid sun damage, follow a healthy lifestyle, develop a protective tan gradually, and avoid burning by wearing a hat and cool-but-covering clothing when out in the strongest sunshine.

Vitamin E

Vitamin E, also known as *alpha tocopherol*, is a **powerful antioxidant**, one of the body's primary defenders against free radical damage to cells and cell membranes. Working with the mineral selenium, it prevents oxidation of fats and cholesterol, so helping to prevent heart disease, cancer and other degenerative problems. It also protects the lungs from damaging air pollutants, and has an important role in maintaining healthy red and also white blood cells.

Sources of vitamin E

Small amounts are widely distributed in many plant foods. Larger amounts come in green, leafy vegetables, unrefined cereals, nuts, seeds, pulses, tofu and sweet potatoes. The richest sources are wheat germ, soya, corn and canola oils and sunflower seeds. Unfortunately heat destroys vitamin E, so cold pressed oils are a better source than refined or processed ones. Animal sources are egg yolks and liver.

Deficiency is rare, because it is so widely available in so many foods.

Toxicity is also rare, as vitamin E is better tolerated than the other fat-soluble vitamins.

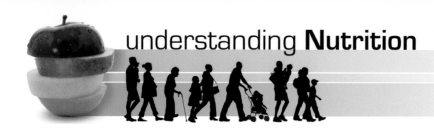
Vitamin K

This is special in that about half of what we need is made by bacteria in the small intestine, from where it is absorbed and stored in the liver. The rest is easily supplied from food.

Function of vitamin K

It is one of the many factors in the cascade of reactions that cause blood to clot. It also has a role in the growth and maintenance of healthy bones.

Food sources of vitamin K

Green, leafy vegetables of the cabbage family are the richest plant source. Smaller but significant amounts are in cereals, fruits and other vegetables. Animal sources are milk, eggs and meat, particularly liver.

Deficiency is possible when drugs interfere with the absorption of vitamin K, or destroy the bacteria that produce it in the gut. Serious deficiency causes uncontrolled bleeding and can be fatal.

Toxicity is rare but can occur from excess supplement use.

Minerals

Minerals are inorganic elements. They do not degenerate or decay with storage or temperature change, and are lost from food only if they are cooked in water, which is then thrown away. We can divide them into major and trace minerals, not according to the importance of their functions but to the amounts in which they are found in the body.

The **major minerals** are calcium, phosphorus, potassium, sulphur, sodium, chlorine and magnesium. These range in quantity from 1200g of calcium and 600g of phosphorus in an average person who weighs 60kg, to magnesium at about 30g, or six teaspoonfuls. There are more than a dozen **trace minerals**, most of their weights measured in milligrams. Iron is the most plentiful and best known, an essential component of the haemoglobin that makes blood red. The average human has about 2.5g or half a teaspoonful of iron. All the minerals are important, whether they are measured in kilos or milligrams, and they are plentiful in both animal foods and unrefined plant foods. Problems begin when foods are refined and minerals are lost, or when heavy use of animal foods upsets the balance. Plant foods contain all the minerals we need in appropriate amounts and in the right combinations.

Calcium is the fifth most plentiful element in the human body, after oxygen, carbon, hydrogen and nitrogen. It accounts for nearly 2% of the body weight, the average adult containing well over a kilo, 99% of which is in the skeleton. Calcium is involved in much of the body's metabolism, which means that the remaining 1% has many important functions. It has roles in the transmission of nerve messages, muscle contraction and relaxation (including the heart muscle), blood pressure control, blood clotting and numerous enzyme and hormone actions. Because these functions are vital to the circulation and nervous system, the blood level of calcium must be kept stable. If the blood level falls, it is immediately replenished by borrowing calcium from the bones, which are not static but very much alive and active. They are being constantly remodelled and the whole skeleton is renewed several times a year.

There is plenty of calcium in food. The best-known source in Europe and America is dairy produce, but what is less well known is that the calcium in dairy produce is not in the most easily absorbed form. Calcium is widely distributed in plant foods like green vegetables, grains, beans, nuts and seeds, mostly in an easily absorbed form. A couple of exceptions are spinach and wheat bran which are both rich in calcium, but in a form that is not easily absorbed. This has given rise to the

myth that calcium is not easily absorbed from plant foods, but it would be a problem only on a restricted diet. A varied whole plant-food diet provides plenty of calcium.

There are several other very important factors in ensuring that there is enough calcium in the body. To absorb calcium into the system, there must be enough vitamin D, the sunshine vitamin. And once the calcium has been absorbed, it is important to limit the factors that cause it to be lost from the body.

In the West, osteoporosis, a degenerative disease characterised by loss of calcium from the bones, is now very common. It has long been thought that the best way to prevent it was with a dairy-rich, high-calcium diet. Interestingly, Europe and America, who

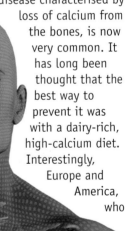

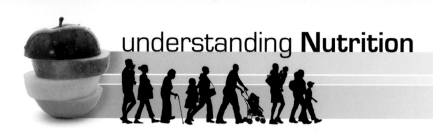

lead the world in calcium intake, also lead the world in osteoporosis. In China, with only a third or a half the calcium intake, people have stronger bones and much less osteoporosis. Evidently calcium intake is not the whole story, and the key factor is not how much you take in but how much of that you lose.

Some of the factors that cause calcium loss are a diet high in animal protein, a high-phosphorus intake from meat and from soft drinks, high salt intake, caffeine, smoking and alcohol, and, very important, lack of exercise. These are all very common in the rich countries of the West. Factors to promote calcium retention are low-protein intake (plant proteins are ideal as they are less concentrated and are lower in phosphorus), low-salt intake, avoiding caffeine, alcohol and phosphorus-rich soft drinks, not smoking and taking regular, vigorous exercise. In China the average person gets far more exercise and eats far less animal produce, two of the most important factors in retaining calcium, and building and keeping healthy bones.

The World Health Organisation recommends 400-500mg of calcium a day for those who do not follow the rich, inactive Western lifestyle. Average intakes in the US and UK are far higher than this, and the UK Food Standards Agency recommends 700mg of calcium a day for adults. Fortunately, there is no need to make detailed dietary assessments: if you are eating a varied diet based on whole, unrefined plant foods, you should have no problem in getting the calcium you need, and, if you get plenty of exercise and avoid the other calcium-lowering factors, you should have no problem in retaining it.

Phosphorus is the next most plentiful mineral. It

60

is a major component of bones and teeth, and in addition it has vital functions in cell membranes, genetic material, maintaining an acid-base balance in the blood and tissues, and energy production. It is highest in animal produce, but is present in so many plants that deficiency is unlikely in almost any diet. However, excess is a distinct possibility if you enjoy animal produce and fizzy drinks, because both are high in phosphorus. When the phosphorus:calcium ratio is too high, the body removes the excess phosphorus, but unfortunately removes calcium from the bones at the same time.

Sulphur: no need to worry about getting enough sulphur as long as you are getting enough food.

At 150g in the body there is plenty of it, mainly in the structure of various proteins. It comes in all protein foods, both plant and animal, as it is part of the structure of a number of amino acids, and is used for building and stabilising proteins in the body. There is so much available in food that there are no known symptoms of deficiency.

Sodium, chlorine and potassium are **electrolytes**, minerals with positive or negative electrical charges. They are vitally important in balancing the amounts and concentrations of the body fluids, both inside and outside the cells and in the blood. In this way they affect the function of every organ and tissue.

Sodium has its main role in the blood and the fluids outside the cells. It maintains fluid balance and is particularly vital in the function of muscles and nerves. It is so plentiful in nature that there is no known diet that lacks it. Excess is common, however, a result of eating too much salt (sodium chloride). Savoury snacks and many processed foods are very high in salt. Animal produce, whether dairy or meat, is also high in sodium. High-sodium intake is associated with high blood pressure, heart attack, stroke and some cancers.

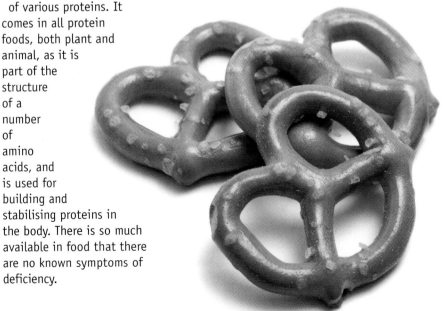

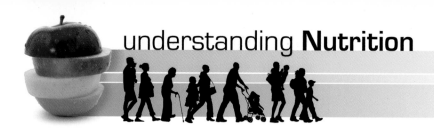

Potassium is the main electrolyte in the fluid inside the cells. It also has critical roles in maintaining fluid balance, and in the function of muscles and nerves. Another of its functions is control of the action of the heart. Fresh fruits and vegetables are the best sources. Deficiency is possible in some illnesses and with the use of some diuretic medicines. Supplements can cause excess which is dangerous too.

Chlorine works with sodium outside the cells, and with potassium inside them. It is abundant in food, and dietary deficiency is rare, but the water and electrolyte balance can be upset by severe vomiting and diarrhoea, and by excessive sweating with dehydration. These conditions call for urgent fluid and electrolyte replacement. Too much salt is dangerous, but too little salt can be fatal, too, which is why marathon runners need to replace electrolytes as well as water.

How much salt do we need?

The Food Standards Agency recommends not more than 6g a day – a teaspoonful. The average person in the UK takes 9.5g a day, and most of this salt comes from processed and packaged food. We can limit salt by avoiding the high-salt snack-foods, choosing home cooking rather than packet soup, sauces and ready meals, and by eating plenty of fruit. Salt makes food taste nice, so the manufacturers act accordingly and add more than we need. Our taste-buds are not a good guide until we have educated them, but they can be re-educated, and once we are used to rather less salt, we won't miss it. On the other hand, it is possible to have too little salt. We lose salt in sweat, so vigorous activity in hot weather may call for extra salt.

Magnesium is the least of the major minerals, at just 30g (or six teaspoonfuls). It is necessary for the operation of hundreds of enzymes. It comes in a very wide range of foods, but particularly good sources are beans, nuts, potatoes, spinach and sunflower seeds. Deficiency has been linked to heart disease, chronic fatigue, depression and many other illnesses.

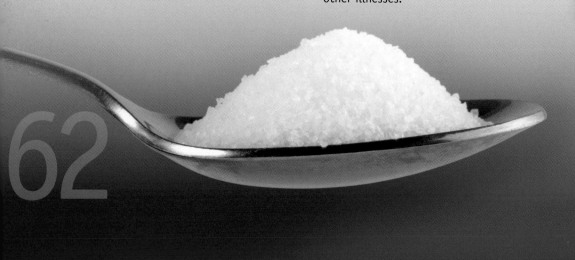

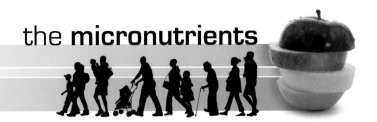

the **micronutrients**

Trace minerals are the ones present in amounts less than 5g (one teaspoonful). Iron is the most plentiful at 2.4g. Though present only in tiny amounts, these trace minerals all have important functions. As well as iron, our bodies use zinc, copper, manganese, iodine, selenium, fluorine, chromium, copper and several other minerals.

Iodine is well known for its relation to the thyroid gland. **Zinc** and **selenium** have multiple functions that involve the immune system and antioxidant activities, making them important in preventing cancer and other degenerative diseases. Most of these trace minerals are widely available in unrefined plant foods and sea salt. Heavy use of refined foods makes deficiencies possible, with important effects on all the body systems. All the trace minerals are toxic in excess. Overuse of supplements is dangerous, underlining the fact that the safest way to get our minerals is from our food.

Iron has a major function in haemoglobin, the oxygen carrying pigment that makes blood red. Most people are aware of the possibility of iron deficiency (anaemia), and it's a worldwide problem. Diseases that cause blood loss are a major factor, as is inadequate iron in the diet, which often simply means inadequate *food*. Most people think that red meat is the most important source of iron, but although plant sources may contain less iron, it is usually in a more easily absorbed form. The richest plant sources are the dark coloured ones, because the iron is in the pigments that give them their dark colour – dark green vegetables, beetroot, prunes, raisins and the dark outer layers of grains. Anaemia is a debilitating condition that most often develops gradually, and although a mineral-rich, whole-food diet is part of the treatment, iron supplements are the quickest way to combat it. It is possible to get excess iron on a meat-rich diet, and it's associated with increased risk of heart disease and other problems.

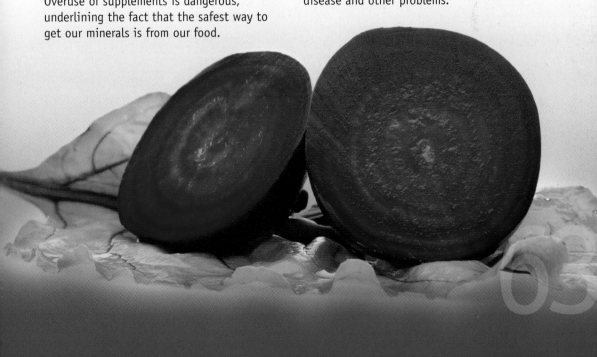

03

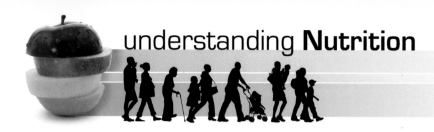

What about mineral supplements?

As with vitamins, people who are or have been unable to get an adequate diet may need mineral supplements. People with certain specific health problems such as anaemia will need them too. In both cases it is wise to get professional advice before taking mineral supplements. For most people, the best 'supplements' are mineral-rich foods. A varied whole-food diet, mainly or entirely vegetarian, is the best defence against mineral deficiencies.

> **A varied whole-food diet, mainly or entirely vegetarian, is the best defence against mineral deficiencies**

Phytochemicals

Why are fruit and vegetables so good for us, that even governments promote them? They are low in fat, low in salt, high in fibre, high in vitamins and minerals, and they contain **phytochemicals**.

These are a huge group of complex substances, present in very tiny amounts, which have only been intensively studied in recent years. The word *phytochemical* simply means plant chemical, but most people use it in a more limited way to mean '*a non-nutritive bioactive substance that has a beneficial effect on human health.*' To put it more simply, phytochemicals are not themselves foods, but they react with our bodies and they do us good.

Phytochemicals are **not nutrients** like the macronutrients that are

Cooking to conserve vitamins and minerals

Food minerals are soluble in water and are easily lost if foods are cooked in water which is thrown away. To avoid this, they should be cooked in as little water as possible and the water should also be used.

Steaming is a good method, especially if the water is saved and used for gravy or soup, or simply consumed as a drink. Stews and soups conserve all the minerals, as do baking and roasting.

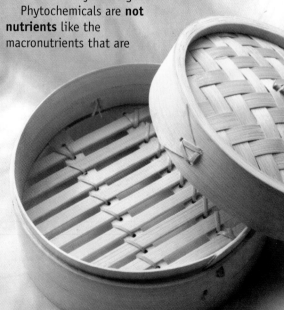

digested, absorbed and used or stored for fuel and other specific functions, nor do they have specific roles in building and maintaining the body and preventing deficiency diseases like the micronutrients.

They are **bioactive** and have a great variety of overlapping biological functions and long-term actions. Because there are so many phytochemicals all working together in harmony, hundreds or even thousands in a single plant food, there are no obvious specific deficiencies, nor are many specific supplements likely to be useful for a long time to come.

Phytochemicals are good for you

They provide the colours, flavours and scents of plants and are also part of their defence system against micro-organisms and other pests. They have very important roles in our defence systems too. They boost our immune systems, and help to prevent heart disease, cancer, other degenerative diseases and ageing generally.

Phytochemicals come in plants

Every edible plant that has been studied so far has a range of these helpful substances. There are many thousands of them, and only relatively few of them have been studied so far. They have a variety of chemical structures and a variety of functions, and any one plant will contain dozens or even hundreds of different ones. But you do not have to be a biochemist to understand their importance.

Phytochemicals belong to a variety of different chemical families such as carotenoids, flavonoids, terpenes and polyphenols. They work in many different ways. Some work as enzymes to speed up the destruction of dangerous cells and organisms. Some are like hormones, as, for example, the phyto-oestrogens in soya beans which seem to block the effect of other oestrogens that could encourage breast and other cancers to develop. Some work at the DNA level, repairing or preventing genetic damage that could lead to cancer. Others work on the cell walls, preventing harmful things from entering. Many other phytochemicals work as enzymes to speed up

65

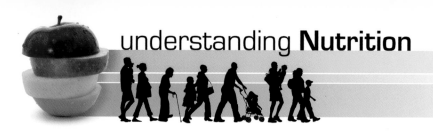

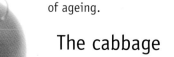

the breakdown of carcinogens and other harmful substances. The largest number work as antioxidants, inactivating the dangerous free radicals that promote cancer, heart disease and other effects of ageing.

The cabbage connection

The first widely publicised anti-cancer plant was the humble cabbage. Epidemiologists had been looking at diets and cancer incidence, and they found that the more cabbage (and other members of the brassica family) in the diet, the lower the incidence of cancer. Studies of the plants themselves showed that they contained many phytochemicals with anti-cancer and anti-ageing properties. (So mothers were right all along when they urged their children to eat their greens!)

Since then all the commonly used plant foods have been studied, and helpful phytochemicals have been found in them all. Thousands have been identified and hundreds of epidemiological studies have confirmed that the more whole plant foods in the diet, the healthier the individual.

Below are a few examples of phytochemicals, where to find them and what they do.

Carotenoids: more than 600 of these have been identified so far. They are the bright yellow, orange and red pigments in carrots, apricots, tomatoes, strawberries, oranges and many other colourful foods, including the dark-green leafy ones, where the green chlorophyll masks the yellow colour. Carotenoids are powerful antioxidants, and also

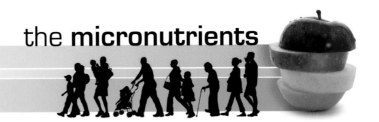

stimulate the immune system and help prevent cancer by regulating genetic activity. Beta-carotene is the best known because it is the precursor of vitamin A.

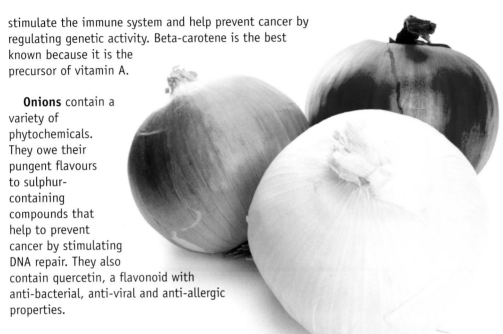

Onions contain a variety of phytochemicals. They owe their pungent flavours to sulphur-containing compounds that help to prevent cancer by stimulating DNA repair. They also contain quercetin, a flavonoid with anti-bacterial, anti-viral and anti-allergic properties.

Garlic, with its bouquet of phytochemicals, helps reduce cholesterol levels, improves blood flow, boosts the immune system and reduces cancer risk. Allicin, the substance that gives garlic its pungent taste and smell, has powerful antibiotic properties, too.

Oranges are loaded with phytochemicals. Nearly two hundred have been studied so far. To protect against cancer, there are 60 flavonoids and 40 liminoids, plus the limonene that gives the distinctive tangy taste to the peel. There are also 20 carotenoids to stimulate the immune system and protect against ageing.

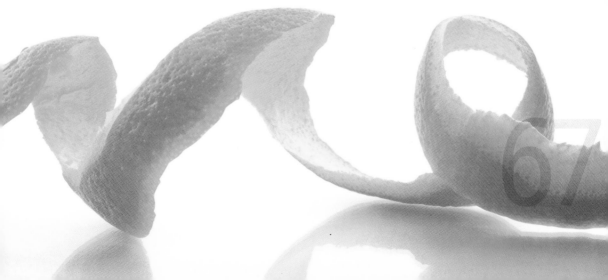

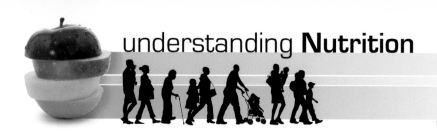

Whole grains are also associated with reduced cancer risk, partly thanks to their phytochemical content, 90% of which is in the bran and germ, and is therefore missing from white flour.

Red grape skins and other red fruit and vegetables contain **resveratrol**, another protective substance which has a special action against oestrogen-dependent and other cancers, and against heart disease. Many think this is an important factor in the benefits of the Mediterranean diet.

Flaxseeds and sesame seeds are rich in **lignans**, which also act against oestrogen and help to prevent breast and prostate cancer. (Remember, flaxseeds are rich in omega 3 oils too.)

Rosemary, sage, thyme, oregano and other kitchen herbs owe their flavours to **terpenoids**, which are strong antioxidants, and also inhibit cholesterol production and have cancer-preventing properties.

Tomatoes contain the health-giving red pigment **lycopene** that has been particularly associated with lowering prostate cancer risk. Interestingly, it is even more available from cooked tomatoes than from raw ones, and it's more easily absorbed if there is oil present, preferably **olive oil**, which contributes its own phenolic phytochemicals to the war on heart disease and cancer. Lycopene is also present in strawberries and many other red fruits and berries.

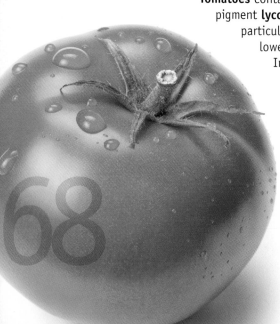

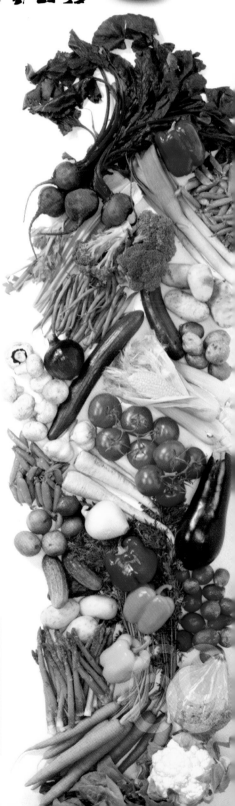

Phytochemicals are often concentrated in the outer parts of plants, like the bran of wheat and the skins of apples – another reason for eating foods in a whole and natural state. This doesn't mean eating everything raw, however. The full complement of phytochemicals may not be released until the cell walls are broken down by cooking, blending or chewing extremely well.

The great thing is that you do not have to know all about phytochemicals in order to benefit from them. The facts are so simple that even a child can understand them.

Summary

Phytochemicals are found in plants. They make plant foods look nice and taste good. They are at their maximum in whole unrefined plant foods. The key word is *variety*.

To maximise your intake of phytochemicals, from day to day eat a wide variety of different coloured plant foods, in as simple, whole and natural a state as possible; some, like grains, always cooked; some, like vegetables, sometimes cooked, sometimes raw.

To get the maximum benefit, enhance your meal with endorphins – the natural calming and cheering chemicals which are produced in your brain when you think thankful thoughts. To do this, before you eat, pause to thank our Creator for giving us these life-enhancing phytochemicals in such beautiful, colourful and delicious packaging. Then eat and enjoy!

The World Cancer Research Fund include tomatoes, peppers, onions, garlic, cabbage, broccoli, Brussels sprouts, carrots, spinach, pumpkinseeds, strawberries, mangos, kiwi fruit, oranges, Brazil nuts and whole-wheat bread in their list of important anti-cancer foods.

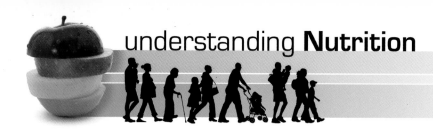
Antioxidants and free radicals

As the body's cells use oxygen to produce energy, they also produce **free radicals.** These are natural by-products of metabolism that cause serious damage if they are allowed to get out of control. Antioxidants are the means of control. Free radicals are unstable molecules which have lost one of their electrons. They replace it by grabbing an electron from another molecule, which grabs from another one and so on, setting up an electron grabbing chain reaction that damages cells and tissues and promotes the degenerative changes that cause ageing and degenerative diseases, including heart disease and cancer.

The 'police' who put a stop to this are the **antioxidants** which seek out the free radicals and inactivate them. Vitamins A, C and E, and many phytochemicals are antioxidants, potent enemies of the dangerous free radicals. For this reason a regular supply of antioxidants is needed, and the best way of ensuring this is to eat a varied, natural, unrefined, plant-food diet.

Here is an easy way to understand **antioxidants** and **free radicals**: Imagine a children's dancing class with all the little boys and girls paired off. While the teacher is out of the room for a moment, an extra boy *(like a free radical)* comes in, and as he has no partner, he grabs the nearest girl. Her partner grabs another girl and soon the room is in an uproar with a rough and noisy game of partner grabbing. The teacher comes back in *(like an antioxidant)* and stops the fun by partnering the last odd boy herself. This rough and noisy game has caused some damage to furniture and fittings *(free radical cell damage)* that must now be repaired, supervised by the teacher *(in another antioxidant-like role)*.

There will always be some free radicals around, because they are a natural product of normal metabolism, just as sparks are a normal product of fires. Problems arise when there are too many free radicals and not enough antioxidants. Radiation, smoking, alcohol and meat are some sources of extra free radicals. A diet rich in plant foods and a balanced lifestyle with adequate exercise and rest ensure a plentiful supply of antioxidants.

Nutrition and specific health problems

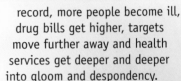

4

The whole Western world is threatened by a vast epidemic of chronic degenerative disease, and health systems everywhere are crushed under its weight. Scientists, sociologists, governments, healthcare providers and many others struggle to discover how to treat the huge burden of disease and suffering. Those who know the causes of the epidemic could be tempted to view many of their efforts as so much rearranging of the deck chairs on the Titanic. As more bodies are set up to investigate, monitor and record, more people become ill, drug bills get higher, targets move further away and health services get deeper and deeper into gloom and despondency.

But there is good news – we know that the main causes of the chronic degenerative diseases are unhealthy lifestyle factors. When the causes are known, prevention is possible. The current epidemic is preventable and many of its effects are reversible. Although it may seem beyond the range of vision of many politicians and planners, we know that healthy lifestyle factors can both prevent chronic degenerative diseases and begin to reverse their effects. Nutrition is a very good place to start.

And what about the rest of the world? The World Health Organisation estimates that up to a sixth of the world's population has inadequate food. Officially, they suffer protein energy malnutrition (PEM). Specific vitamin deficiencies complicate the picture. PEM has a particularly devastating effect on children, stunting both physical and mental development. Malnutrition also depresses the immune system in both adults and children, diminishing their ability to fight infectious diseases. The poorest countries have a double burden:

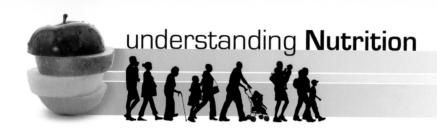

their poorest citizens weakened by diseases due to hunger, and their more prosperous citizens at risk of the degenerative diseases due to excess.

Obesity, high blood pressure and high blood cholesterol

These are not themselves diseases, but are important precursors of chronic degenerative diseases. Unhealthy lifestyles are responsible, and the rich Western diet with its excesses of fat, sugar and animal protein is often the most important factor. Changing to a diet based on natural whole plant foods, getting enough exercise, avoiding poisons and cultivating an optimistic outlook are the best ways to avoid or reverse these conditions and the problems to which they lead. Obesity increases the risk and severity of all these problems. Winning the battle against obesity is vital to the success of the war against degenerative disease.

Nutrition – a key to all degenerative problems

All our cells need oxygen, water and food, with vitamins, minerals and phytochemicals. They need an efficient transport system to deliver them and to remove waste products. The blood is the transport medium, and if it's thick and viscous and the arteries are

clogged with fatty material, the cells and tissues go short of the oxygen and nutrients they need. This causes the tissues to degenerate and this is the process whereby degenerative diseases start. Lack of oxygen and proper nutrition causes tissues to age prematurely, resulting in many different diseases, depending on each individual's strengths and weaknesses. In some it will be arthritis first, in others, coronary artery disease, in others, cancer.

Coronary artery disease and other circulatory problems

Key factors in these diseases are narrowed arteries and blood that clots too easily. The Western diet is a major contributor. Diets high in animal fat raise the blood cholesterol to levels where fat is deposited in arteries and blood becomes viscous. Gradually, over the course of a life, the arteries clog up with fatty material, setting the scene for heart attacks, strokes and other problems. Whole plant foods promote healthy hearts and arteries. This is because they are low in fat and sugar and high in fibre and antioxidants. They also contain phytochemicals, and these factors work together to thin the blood and keep the arteries clean and strong.

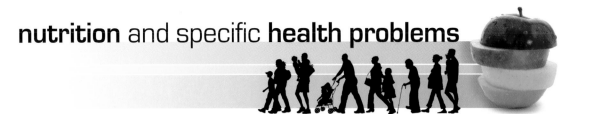

Cancer

The term cancer covers a large group of diseases where the immune system has failed and allows certain kinds of damaged cells to grow out of control.

There is good news: most cancer is preventable! Apart from tobacco and lung cancer, fifty years ago the cause of most cancers was still pretty much a mystery to most people, lay and medical alike. The situation is quite different now. Not only is tobacco universally recognised as being responsible for many cancer deaths, but we now have much more knowledge about the many other factors that work together to produce this dreaded disease. Conservative authorities claim that 30% of all cancers are due to avoidable environmental causes. Others would put the figure nearer to

80% for the number of cancers due to avoidable factors (many of them dietary) – in other words, to unhealthy lifestyle choices. This really is good news, because although cancer is more than twice as common as it was in the 1950s, *we now have the choice whether or not to take personal action to lower our own risk of developing 'the big C'.* This is not just true of the West. Recent World Health Reports show a steady increase in cancer incidence in developing countries, as more and more of their populations adopt Western lifestyles.

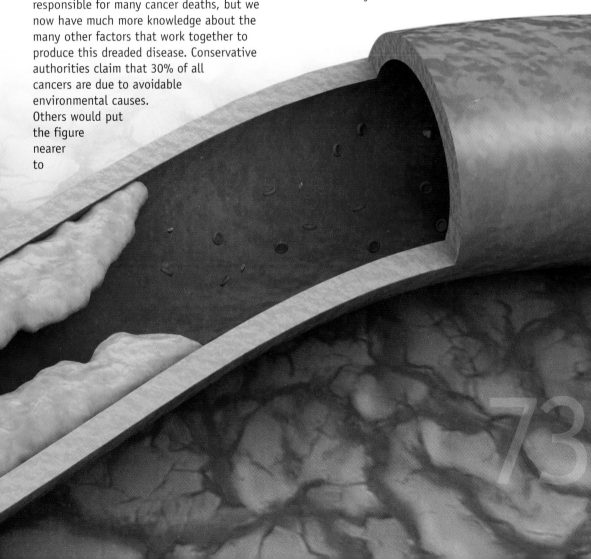

73

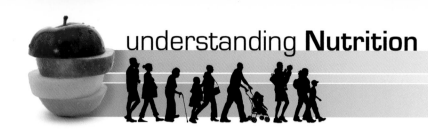

Cancer-promoting factors to avoid

Food: epidemiologists studying the relationship of cancer to lifestyle in many different societies have concluded that a high-animal-fat intake promotes cancer. Studies found that breast cancer was low in Japan, but high in Japanese immigrants to the United States. Careful study showed that the important difference was the change from the low-fat, mainly plant food with fish Japanese diet, to the typical refined, high-fat, high-meat-and-dairy-content Western diet.

Obesity: another result of the Western diet and lifestyle is itself a risk factor for cancer, particularly the common reproductive and digestive-system types.

Other factors: tobacco and alcohol are also very important factors, as are stress and lack of exercise. Radiation, toxic chemicals, food additives, and so on, do play a part, but it is far less important than the factors listed above.

There are *two lines of defence* which, for most people, will help prevent most cancers from starting: *avoiding cancer-promoting factors and choosing cancer-suppressing ones.* And for those who already have cancer these two lines of defence will strengthen their immune systems to give them the very best chance of recovery.

Preventive factors to practise

Food: *eat more fruit and vegetables.* They strengthen the immune system to fight cancer. Eat less refined food and animal produce; ideally, phase them out completely, and *choose to eat unrefined plant foods with their full quota of cancer-preventing vitamins and phytochemicals.*

Other factors
Exercise, sunlight in moderation, rest, healthy reaction to stress, an optimistic outlook, are all important immune-system boosters.
Good medical care is important too, and this is another area where we should be informed and observant, reporting any unusual or persistent and unexplained symptoms promptly, so they can be checked out and swift action taken if needed.

Diabetes

This disease, characterised by uncontrolled blood sugar, is increasing alarmingly in all the

74

developed countries and wherever else Western diets and lifestyles are common. It, too, is a preventable, and, in many cases, a reversible disease. The rich food and sedentary lifestyle, so much desired by those who know the pangs of hunger and exhaustion, unfortunately lead to the chronic degenerative diseases of civilisation, including diabetes and many others.

There are two major types of diabetes. Though they have similarities, they are two different diseases. **Type 1** begins as an acute and very serious illness, most often in children or young people. The pancreas fails to produce insulin and they need regular insulin injections to stay alive. This is **Type 1** or **Insulin Dependent Diabetes Mellitus (IDDM)**

Much more common is **Type 2**, or **Non-Insulin Dependent Diabetes Mellitus (NIDDM)**, which usually develops gradually over many years. It is related to diet and lifestyle. The rich, high-fat, high-sugar Western diet, and the inactive Western behaviour are the chief culprits. This used to be known as 'maturity onset diabetes', but not any more. This is because over the past few years, as calorie intake has increased and activity has decreased, Type 2 diabetes is now occurring in teenagers and even children. As either type of diabetes progresses, *serious complications* develop – heart and arterial disease, kidney failure and blindness. Medical treatment can slow their development and early interventions can reduce and postpone some of the worst effects, but they do not cure.

The real answer to NIDDM is a programme to halt and then to reverse the disease process. Such a programme exists and has been successfully put into practice many thousands of times. It is so simple that most NIDDM patients can manage it by themselves at home, with the minimum of medical monitoring. **IDDM patients will benefit too.** They won't be able to restore their lost insulin production so they won't be able to stop their injections or escape all medical supervision, but their diabetes will become easier to control, complications will be less severe, their general health will improve and they will be more in control of their lives.

So what is this wonderful programme and how does it work? Just as NIDDM is caused mainly by too much of the wrong kind of food and too little exercise, **exercise and right eating can start the healing process.**

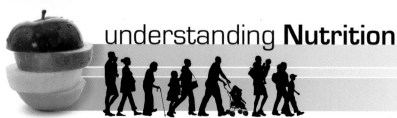

Right eating: the low-calorie, low-sugar, low-fat, wholesome, *unrefined plant-food diet is the answer.* To reverse the disease processes, it is necessary to eat only as many calories as the body requires, and to ensure that those calories come from 100% nutritious food that contains all the micronutrients needed for restoring and healing the damaged tissues. This is the diet based on unrefined starches (wholemeal bread and other unrefined cereal products), vegetables, fruits, nuts and seeds (beans, lentils, and so on). Meal-timing is important, too, as it is best to eat at regular times, and with the main meals at the times when their energy is needed for the day's activities. This means a big breakfast and lunch and a light evening meal.

Exercise: the right amount of exercise for most can be as simple as a half-hour brisk walk twice a day.

Other factors like abstinence from poisons, a regular daily programme, and a cheerful, thankful mental attitude are very important too.

Osteoporosis

Osteoporosis ('porous bone') is a disease which silently and at first painlessly affects the bones. They gradually become thinner and more fragile until the middle of the bone is soft, spongy, and easily broken.

This is very common in the West, and affects mainly older women. The first sign of the disease is often a fracture of the hip, wrist or vertebra. Hip fractures are the most disabling, but vertebral fractures, although often painless at the time, can also be disabling. Multiple vertebral fractures can cause from two to eight inches of height loss, with consequent disability.

Things which increase the risk of osteoporosis for both sexes include a sedentary lifestyle, smoking, caffeine, alcohol, and **a high-protein, high-saturated fat, low-fruit-and-vegetable diet.**

A high-protein diet causes calcium to be leached out of the bones and lost in the urine. Calcium has many vital roles in our bodies, and if our intake is low our bodies may need to take calcium out of the bones, laying the foundation for osteoporosis.

How to maintain calcium levels

The high-calcium content of milk

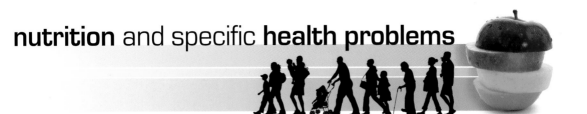

has received much media attention and many people think that dairy produce is essential for the maintenance of calcium levels and healthy bones. However, in milk the calcium is combined with protein, which causes calcium *loss*. While other factors undoubtedly play a part, it is interesting to note that osteoporosis is most common in countries where the consumption of dairy products is high, and rare where it is low.

A lower protein diet helps. Plant proteins are more alkaline and contain less sodium and sulphur than animal proteins, and this also reduces calcium loss. They are also naturally associated with fibre which is filling, and so reduces the chance of eating too much protein anyway. A well-balanced, whole-food vegetarian diet will provide for all your calcium needs.

Food allergies and sensitivities

Allergies are becoming much more common. In some areas, over 30% of 13- and 14-year-olds complain of asthma, and 40% of hay fever, and health services struggle to keep up. Is the answer a crash programme of training new allergists, or are there simpler (and cheaper) solutions, perhaps involving food?

An allergy is a hypersensitivity of the immune system to a foreign substance, such as pollen, house dust or particular foods, which are harmless to non-allergic people. The over-reactive immune system treats these normally harmless substances as invaders, going into emergency mode with the well-known allergic responses of wheezing (asthma), running nose (allergic rhinitis or hay-fever), and skin problems (eczema, urticaria or nettle rash), and, in

77

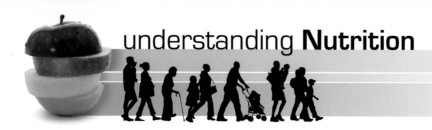

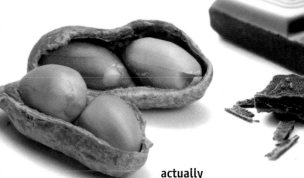

extreme cases, anaphylactic shock – a very dangerous, potentially fatal, condition. Some people have a much greater tendency to these reactions than others, and their condition is known as **atopy**. Most cases of atopy involve many factors, including foods, but the term 'food allergy' is also used very widely for all sorts of reactions to foods, many of which are not allergies at all. For these the term **food sensitivity** is better.

Both true food allergies and other food sensitivities are much more common now than they were twenty or thirty years ago. This is especially so with nut allergy, particularly peanut allergy, where a potentially fatal reaction to this normally harmless nut can occur within minutes. Unfortunately, such severe reactions are very much less rare than they were.

Why is this so? Many people now have unstable immune systems which overreact, like a burglar alarm set to call the police when burglars enter but which, in fact, goes off when a spider walks past. Instead of producing a few drops of fluid to flush out some pollen grains, these over-reactive immune systems produce a torrent of hay-fever or a severe attack of wheezing. Research is needed to find out why so many people's immune systems are so jumpy. Theories range from immune-system overload due to the vast number of foreign chemicals to which we are exposed now, to immune-system *under*-activity, due to our over-hygienic environment. Another possible cause is that immunisation programmes have wiped out the childhood illnesses that helped to build healthy immune responses in the past. Probably all these factors play a part, but the fact is that we do not really know.

Although we do not fully understand food allergies and sensitivities, we do know that **improving general health, lifestyle and environment can greatly diminish, if not** actually **completely cure, many of these problems**. Smoke-free air for asthma sufferers is an obvious example, and pollen-free air for hay-fever sufferers is another. What is less well known is that **asthma and other atopic sufferers can be helped very much by changing their diet**. The same is true for those who find that specific food sensitivities cause problems as diverse as digestive upsets, sinusitis, chronic fatigue, irritable nerves, and even arthritis.

Frequently used foods are the most likely culprits – such well-trusted staples as milk, bread, chocolate, and even orange juice. In the West most people have grown up to look on **milk** as almost the ideal form of nutrition, but it can cause major problems. Actually, as many as **90% of adults worldwide lack the enzymes needed to digest cow's milk**. Milk-production methods have changed a lot over the past decades, too, as has the food industry. With milk in some form added to almost every processed food you can think of, many people are getting milk overload. Milk sensitivity contributes to the truly allergic (atopic) problems and also to most ear, nose and throat troubles, as well as a great many bowel disorders. After milk, the second most common problem food seems to be **wheat**. It's another frequently eaten food, and people now eat less of other cereals, such as oats, rye,

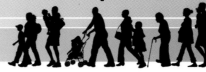

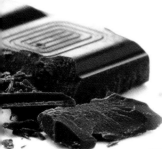

As milk is the commonest problem food, the first step would be to eliminate it and all its products as completely as possible

barley, or rice, to balance it. It's as if the body finally gets wheat overload and goes on strike. There are now very few varieties of wheat grown and this may well add to the problems.

Another problem group is the methyl xanthenes (natural flavourings) – they are in **tea, coffee, chocolate and cola** – another type of substance that many people use daily, or more often than is wise.

Such foods increase the tendency to true allergic or atopic reactions, but acute reactions are often triggered by other less frequently used items which are usually fairly easy to recognise, such as seafood, mushrooms, specific fruits – strawberry is a well-known one – and, of course, the notorious peanut. Sometimes a particular combination of foods, environmental factors and one's mental state is necessary to trigger such reactions, which makes detection much more difficult.

So what should one do? **Those who have experienced severe reactions should, of course, be under medical care, avoid the obvious causes and have medication for emergency use.** They should continue this regime but also start a lifestyle programme to stabilise and strengthen their immune systems. Such a programme includes exercise and stress control as well as a healthy diet. Those with less serious problems will benefit from such a programme too, and it's well worth trying a simple elimination diet to find out what their main triggers are.

from the diet, preferably for a few weeks. If that works, try a 'challenge' – a serving of dairy produce. If the sneezing, bowel cramps or other symptoms recur, the best plan is to avoid all dairy produce for two or three months. After that, many people find they can tolerate it occasionally, sometimes even regularly. The same can be done with wheat, methyl xanthenes and whatever food they suspect. If they are really keen, they can try eliminating dairy, wheat, chocolate, and so on, all at the same time, then reintroduce them gradually one by one to see which ones cause problems.

Eliminating irritating foods is not the whole story however. They need to be replaced by **a wide variety of whole and healthy foods**. Base your diet around unrefined starches, add plenty of fruit and vegetables, and smaller helpings of foods made from beans, nuts and seeds. Eat a wide variety of foods from day to day, but a small variety at any one meal. Avoid eating between meals or late at night. Exercise is very important, too, as is avoiding poisons. **Cultivating a peaceful and contented frame of mind** may be the most important remedy of all.

79

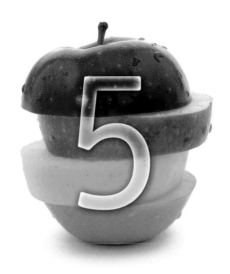

Weight control

There is now a world epidemic of obesity. The USA leads the world, with the majority of its population overweight. Britain is the fattest country in the EU and is fast catching up with the USA. Even poor countries are facing this problem. Their richer citizens are as prone to obesity as the West, and the problem will increase as more and more people aspire to and achieve the Western lifestyle, with its lack of exercise and its abundance of fattening food.

Overweight is a serious problem because it predisposes the individual to a vast range of diseases. Some of these diseases, for example, hernias and varicose veins, are simply due to the extra volume of fat itself. Some, like osteoarthritis, are due to the excess wear and tear the extra weight puts on the spine, hips and knees. Others, like gall stones, diabetes, coronary heart disease and stroke, are due to the changes obesity produces in the body chemistry. Life-threatening illnesses are not only more common, but are more often fatal in the overweight. Even cancer, including some of the commonest types such as breast, colon and prostate, is associated with excess weight. Clearly, being the right weight is very important for health as well as beauty. If you put health first and weight second, you will find that the weight eventually normalises, but it just doesn't seem to work the other way round. In the long run, adequate exercise and a positive, cheerful outlook are as important as diet for good health and lasting weight control. Achieving the right weight has to be part of an ongoing life plan and not just an isolated scheme for a few weeks or months. 'I must lose weight for the holidays' is not the motivation for lasting success!

Being the right weight involves the whole person, not just his eating habits.

The first thing in weight control is to come to terms with one's body type, and then to concentrate on getting healthy, because optimum health will ultimately lead to the right weight. Many people are unhappy with their bodies, not appreciating the wonder of the overall design and the variations that are normal. Some are designed to be below average weight, some above, but definitely none is intended to be obese. Some people do put on weight much more easily than others. Their metabolism is very economical, and they burn less energy and have extra left over to store. Others have a different metabolism that tends to burn at a higher rate, and they just never seem to get fat, no matter what they eat. Actual endocrine disturbances, for example thyroid deficiency, that

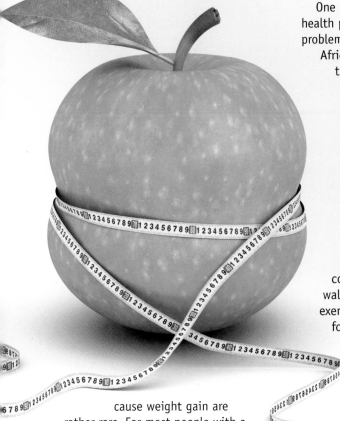

cause weight gain are rather rare. For most people with a weight problem, the solution is not medication but dedication!

If you want to maximise your health, it is absolutely essential to be in control of what you eat. You cannot allow the taste, sight or remembrance of a food to dictate what you eat. Many weight-control programmes fail because they do not retrain your thinking about food. Clearly, if you make an enormous effort to exercise self-discipline and deny yourself cream cakes and chocolate, you may lose weight, but continue to think longingly of them, and you are unlikely to resist the urge to eat them when you have reached your goal. Sadly, if that's the case, as so many can testify, your weight won't stay down.

One of the most important parts of any health plan is **exercise**. Weight is not a problem for the Masai tribesmen in East Africa, who spend all day on the run with their cattle, or with the Hunza in Northern Pakistan who walk up and down mountains all day. We are designed to be active, not to be sitting all day, and we are at our best when we get vigorous activity. One reason why some people do not lose weight, even on the most frugal diets, is that exercise is necessary to stimulate the body to burn up the calories and to activate the appetite-control centre in the brain. *Regular* exercise is vital for weight control, not a sport once a week or a walk on Sundays, but regular *daily* exercise. Few exercises can beat walking, for safety and convenience. Several miles a day would be good, with a gradual increase in speed and duration. No time for exercise? Take the long-term view. The investment of time in daily exercise from now on may add several extra years of healthy life. And, incidentally, it is the exercise you enjoy that does you the most good, so find something you really like doing.

For good health and weight control you need to eat the **right amount** of the **right**

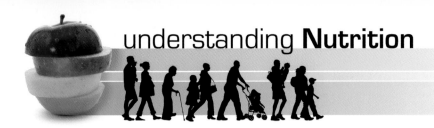
kind of food at the **right time** in the **right frame of mind**.

You stay the same weight when the energy in the food you eat equals the energy you use up. Clearly, if the energy output is low and the food intake is high, there's going to be a surplus to be stored away as fat. This is the case with the typical high-fat Western diet, in which 40-45% of the calories come from fat, and as much as 80-90% of the food may be refined. Most slimming diets try to solve the problem by reducing the food intake to below the supposed energy output so that the stored fat is mobilised and used up. Unfortunately, these low-calorie diets are unsatisfying and demand more will power than most people have. If the food intake is really low, the body goes into starvation mode, conserving every possible calorie, breaking down muscle tissue as well as fat, endangering health, and making weight loss very difficult.

The right kind of food

The right amount is the amount needed to satisfy hunger, rather than appetite, but most people in the developed countries do not really know what hunger is. Choosing the **right kind** of food makes it much easier to eat the right amount. **Whole-plant foods** are more bulky, so one feels fuller and more satisfied. These foods have their full complement of vitamins and minerals, and they do not contain excess calories. Refined foods have less bulk, are less filling, and have more calories. Excess calorie intake is almost inevitable when these foods form a large part of the diet. In addition, they are deficient in the vitamins, minerals and phytochemicals that the body needs to metabolise all those calories and to fight disease. Their absence creates even more dissatisfaction and sometimes cravings and addictions as well. Eating very

The more natural the food, the more fibre it is likely to contain and the more filling it is. Soft, smooth foods like ice-cream or chocolate mousse go down very quickly and are not very satisfying. White bread, as well as being less filling, has more calories – two good reasons to choose whole-wheat bread. Here is another example: about ten raw apples have the same number of calories as one piece of apple pie with ice-cream. Raw apples are much more filling. Who could possibly want to chew his way through more than five? But a person could well have a double helping of pie and ice-cream.

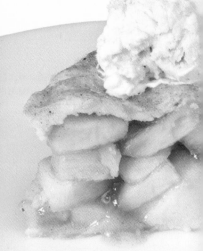

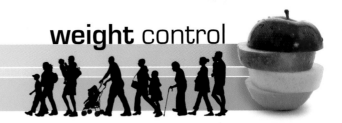

quickly also leads to overeating, whereas eating slowly, savouring each mouthful and chewing it well, increases the level of satisfaction.

> **Two dangerous dietary myths that need to be exploded**
> *'High-protein diets are the way to lose weight.'* While it is true that the metabolism of protein uses extra energy and that high-protein diets can result in rapid weight loss, it's at a price. High protein intake puts stress on the liver, kidneys and heart.
> *'Starchy foods like bread and potatoes are fattening.'* Unrefined starchy foods are filling and prevent overeating, so the opposite is true, though of course bread becomes fattening when thickly spread with butter, as do potatoes when they are made into chips.

Fat provides more than twice as many calories as carbohydrate and protein, so it makes sense to eat less of it, but in itself fat is not bad. In the right amount, as found in natural, unrefined plant foods, it is good. Some is necessary to enable us to absorb the fat-soluble vitamins – and it adds flavour and interest to the diet. A varied diet of unrefined plant foods is not a fat-free diet, and need not even be a very low-fat diet. There is plenty of healthy natural fat in nuts, seeds, olives and avocados. It's not these (in moderate amounts) that cause the problems; it's the *added* fats. A very overweight person would be wise to be careful not to use too much of even natural high-fat foods, but few should cut them out completely without expert advice.

The food industry and low-fat food

The food industry has had great success with the sale of low-fat food, but it has actually been found that we get fatter when we use these foods. This is because fat gives a feeling of satisfaction, limiting the intake. What happens is that we eat larger amounts of the low-fat foods; the total number of calories is higher, so the weight goes up. Low-fat sweet things are extra high in sugar. Low-fat spreads may not be of much help either, especially if we eat them in double the quantity of the old full-fat spreads.

83

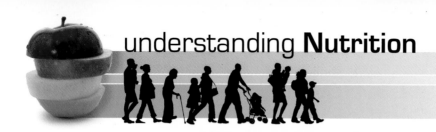

What about animal products?

Even apart from the question of the association of animal foods with degenerative disease, they are not the best for a weight-reducing diet, because they tend to be concentrated foods, high in calories, fat and protein. If they are used, it should be in small amounts, the main part of the diet being a variety of whole-plant foods with a basis of unrefined starches, and plenty of fruit and vegetables.

What about drinks?

They can be your worst enemies in the battle for weight control. Fizzy soft drinks are mainly sugared water. Alcoholic drinks are even worse, because alcohol itself is not a food, but a rich source of empty calories. Even natural fruit juices are high in calories. **The best drink for weight control is water.** Tea and coffee do not contain calories, unless you add sugar, milk or cream, but caffeine is a drug with withdrawal effects, one of which is a feeling of let-down that can be confused with hunger, which makes appetite control more difficult.

What about counting calories?

Not a good idea! If we choose a varied, unrefined, mainly plant-food diet, there is no need for this tedious exercise. The principle is to eat enough healthy food to feel

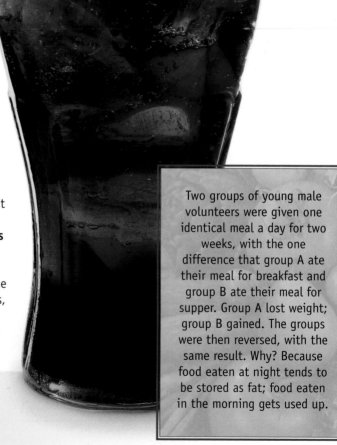

Two groups of young male volunteers were given one identical meal a day for two weeks, with the one difference that group A ate their meal for breakfast and group B ate their meal for supper. Group A lost weight; group B gained. The groups were then reversed, with the same result. Why? Because food eaten at night tends to be stored as fat; food eaten in the morning gets used up.

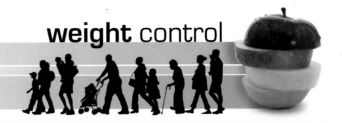

satisfied, and to exercise enough to raise our metabolism sufficiently to burn it up.

Does it matter *when* we eat?

Very much so. A regular programme is one of the secrets of appetite and weight control. *A large, filling breakfast* will set you up for the day and eliminate the need for between meal snacks (which are usually high-fat or high-sugar). *If you make a decision not to eat between meals*, you will save yourself the trouble of having to make a decision every time you are tempted. Another reason for a good breakfast is that food eaten in the morning tends to be burned up during the course of the day's activities.

Summary: eat a big breakfast, a moderate lunch and a small evening meal. The old adage: 'Breakfast like a king, lunch like a prince, sup like a pauper' is especially valid for those who are battling with their weight. Those who are seriously overweight would be wise to miss evening meals altogether.

The frame of mind in which we eat is important too. It's very easy to eat for emotional reasons. Lonely and sad people who feel rejected often eat for comfort, and, unfortunately, comfort foods are usually high in sugar and fat. Self-respect and self-acceptance are healthy emotions at mealtimes, along with acceptance of the laws of life and a thankful heart. It's vital to cultivate interests in subjects other than food, and to take an active interest in other people and their problems as well as one's own.

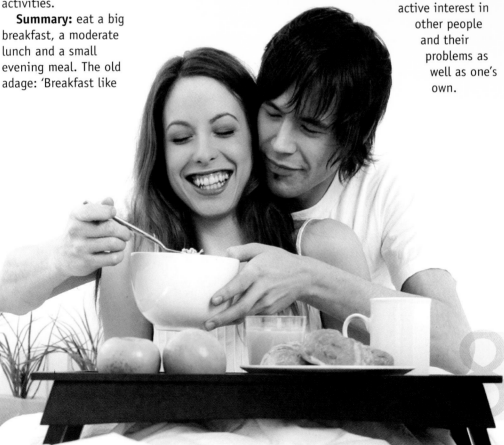

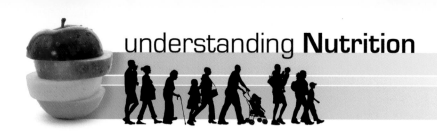

The long-term view is best

Improving one's health, or correcting one's weight each needs to be a long-term project. Usually it has taken years to gain the excess weight, and the best way is to reduce it slowly, sometimes over several years. Many popular diets aim at a loss of two pounds (nearly 2 kg) a week, but a steady half-pound a week adds up to an impressive 26 pounds in a year. The diet and lifestyle changes that are made gradually will be easier to maintain, unlike the usual slimming diet with its promised quick results but short-lived success. The healthy lifestyle needs to be *lifelong*.

What motivation is needed for a lasting change of lifestyle and eating habits? Gratitude to our Creator for designing our bodies for maximum enjoyment of life, and our food for maximum health and eating pleasure is the best motivation for a long-term change.

An important note about exercise!

Exercise helps to control the appetite. It increases the metabolic rate so calories burn faster, and this continues for several hours after the exercise is over. It helps the heart and circulation, the digestion, the immune system, the mood. Appropriate exercise benefits every part of the human system, so must be an important part in every health-promoting programme. In order to be really effective, exercise should be enjoyable, and do not forget that walking is the simplest, safest and best form of exercise for most people.

Choices

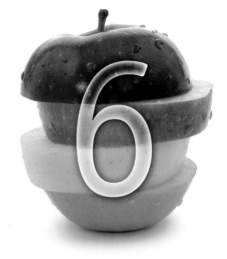

To eat or not to eat meat?

How does meat eating contribute to the epidemic of degenerative disease that is ravaging the rich industrialised countries?

Saturated fat and cholesterol are two of the problems, especially where diseases of the heart and circulation are concerned. Cholesterol, the fatty material that blocks the arteries, is much more likely to be deposited there if saturated fat is present.

All foods of animal origin contain cholesterol because it's part of the structure of all animal cells, including ours. Our bodies are able to manufacture all they need and to deal with small amounts in the diet, but we do not *need* to eat it at all.

Animal foods tend to be high in saturated fats. This is especially true of the large meat animals, cows, sheep, pigs and all their products. Birds and fish have more of the unsaturated fats and this is why many health authorities advise reducing the intake of red meat (or at least cutting off the fat) and eating more fish and poultry instead. But they all contain cholesterol, which is still a problem, even when the saturated fat is reduced or absent.

No plant contains any cholesterol at all. It just isn't a part of plant cells. **And the majority of plant fats are unsaturated.**

Plant foods contain **fibre**. Fibre keeps everything moving smoothly along the digestive tract, taking all sorts of possibly harmful things out of the body with it, including excess cholesterol, thereby helping to prevent heart disease and many other problems, including bowel cancer.

Animal foods have no fibre of this kind whatsoever.

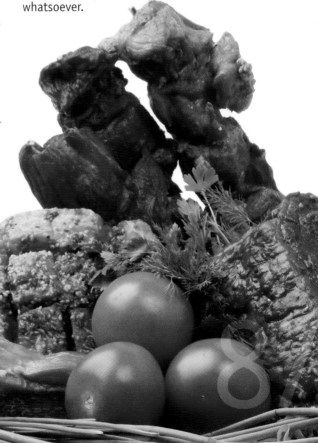

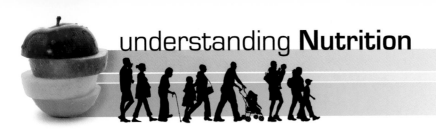

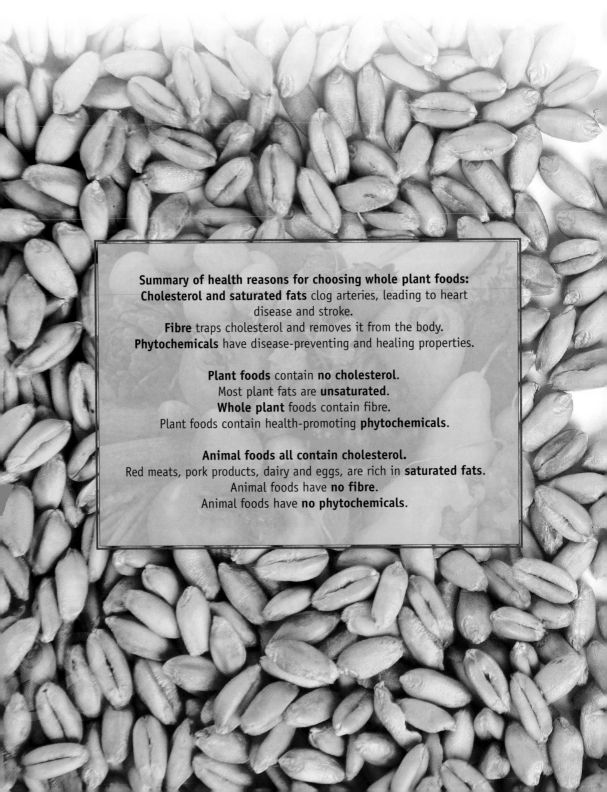

Summary of health reasons for choosing whole plant foods:
Cholesterol and saturated fats clog arteries, leading to heart disease and stroke.
Fibre traps cholesterol and removes it from the body.
Phytochemicals have disease-preventing and healing properties.

Plant foods contain **no cholesterol**.
Most plant fats are **unsaturated**.
Whole plant foods contain fibre.
Plant foods contain health-promoting **phytochemicals**.

Animal foods all contain cholesterol.
Red meats, pork products, dairy and eggs, are rich in **saturated fats**.
Animal foods have **no fibre**.
Animal foods have **no phytochemicals**.

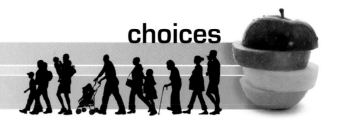

Animals can also transmit their own infectious diseases to humans. The BSE scare has faded from most memories: a very rare but very nasty degenerative disease of the nervous system, apparently transmitted through eating meat contaminated with nervous-system tissues from affected cows. Poultry and eggs are frequently contaminated by salmonella, and most food-handling regulations are about preventing the spread of bacteria from animal foods to humans. There are also numerous parasites that can be transmitted by undercooked meat. Animals also get cancer, but the length of time the disease takes to develop makes the animal connection more difficult to prove. However, epidemiological studies link higher cancer incidence with meat eating.

Thankfully, people do not get plant diseases. Plants can transmit diseases only if contaminated from elsewhere, for example, in salads by salmonella from uncooked chicken, or spoiled – some sorts of mould can cause cancer – and, of course, some plants are poisonous, but then they aren't foods.

Many scientific papers have demonstrated the association between animal fat, cholesterol, and heart disease – going back fifty or more years. The research papers would fill a large room from floor to ceiling.

Epidemiological research (studying the incidence of disease in different groups) shows very clearly that degenerative diseases, particularly heart disease and cancer, are associated with high-animal-fat intake.

The Adventist Health Study is one of the most interesting – read about it in Appendix 1 (page 109).

Meat is very uneconomical to produce. In a world where overpopulation and malnutrition threaten to be major problems in the next few decades, a plant food diet holds the only reasonable promise of a solution. In a world threatened by global warming and water shortages, it's interesting to read that the United Nations Food and Agriculture Organisation reported in 2006 that almost a fifth of climate-changing greenhouse gases comes from the livestock industry. Livestock farming also consumes vast quantities of water, is a major reason for deforestation, and when both pasture and feed production are included, they estimate that it occupies 30% of the earth's usable surface – about ten times as much as would an equal amount of plant foods. A whole plant food diet is healthier, more economical, better for the environment and much better for the animals. This is a case where all the arguments seem to fit together – as if they were all part of some great design. That, in fact, is exactly the situation. Human beings are designed to eat plant foods. There is an overall divinely ordained plan – nature is rational, not chaotic.

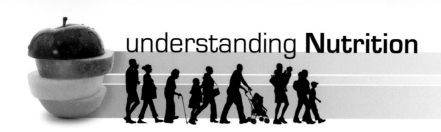

What about eggs, milk and other dairy produce?

Eggs first

Eggs are a very concentrated food, and their yolks are the richest known source of cholesterol. If you can guarantee that the hens are healthy and are fed on healthy food, and you are healthy yourself, and on an otherwise plant-based diet, one or two eggs a week are acceptable. Unfortunately, modern egg-production methods do not guarantee these things, and eggs are associated with the same health problems as meat and dairy produce.

Now for milk

Cow's milk is quite different from human milk, as you would expect if you remember that a cow reaches its full size in a couple of years, compared to a human who takes a great deal longer. To supply the needs of the growing calf, cow's milk is higher in protein, has plenty of cholesterol and contains a lot of growth hormone. Only humans drink the milk of another species and only humans drink milk when they are grown up.

Milk and degenerative disease

The societies which use the most dairy produce also have the highest rates of chronic degenerative disease, and there is a direct relationship between the amounts of dairy produce in the diet and the incidence of the reproductive-system cancers, including breast and prostate cancer. Research in the laboratory confirms the relationship between the growth and other hormones in milk and these cancers.

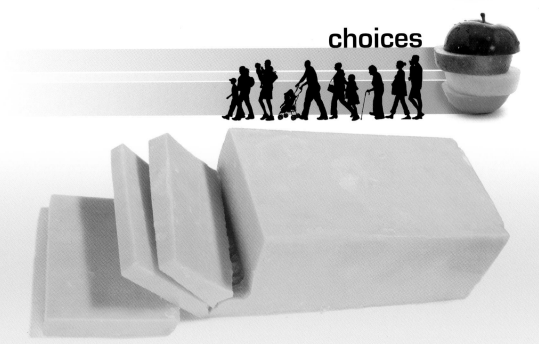

Milk and allergies

The majority of allergies involve milk and can be helped by a dairy-free diet.

Milk and ear, nose and throat problems

Milk sensitivity is a factor in most catarrhal problems, including ear infections in children, sinusitis and chronic running noses.

Milk and the digestive system

About 90% of adults lack sufficient lactase to digest the lactose in milk. (Most of the 10% are in the Western countries which depend on the dairy industry.) This means that they cannot digest dairy foods properly, and suffer with uncomfortable bowel symptoms. Most people with irritable bowel problems are probably short of lactase and can be helped by a dairy-free diet.

Milk and obesity

Much of dairy produce is high in fat and calories generally – butter, cheese, cream, ice-cream and all the appealing foods made with these things. Controlling weight is easier without them.

Milk and pollutants

Milk is highly nutritious, so it's an ideal place for bacteria and other organisms to grow, some from the cow itself, some from outside, and they are not all destroyed by pasteurisation. Other potential problems are caused by antibiotics and other drugs given to the cows.

Milk and animal welfare

The dairy industry is closely linked to the meat industry, and most cows have short and unnaturally hard lives, which gives animal lovers another reason to choose a plant-food diet.

Cream, butter and cheese

Fresh cream is the best of these: it's the least concentrated and the easiest to digest. Butter is next as it is such a concentrated fat. Hard cheeses (like cheddar) are the worst, because not only are they a very concentrated form of dairy produce, but during the fermentation process some undesirable chemical processes occur, which make them harder to digest and, in the long term, more likely to damage the arteries and contribute to cancer. One of these chemical processes is the oxidation of the cholesterol, which makes it much more likely to be deposited in the arteries. Soft cheeses are light and easy to digest and do not contain the harmful chemicals that are produced by the ageing process.

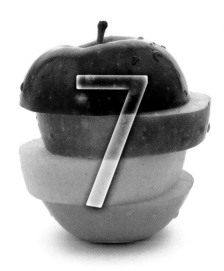

Making the transition to a healthier diet

From the ordinary Western diet

This diet is what a great many people all over the world eat. It's high in refined carbohydrate, refined vegetable oil and animal produce, with 40% or more of the calories coming from fat, some of it saturated fat from animal sources, most of the rest from refined vegetable oils. Much of the carbohydrate is refined sugar and most of the rest is refined cereal. Most of the protein is from animal sources. This is the diet that sets the scene for the current epidemic of obesity and leads to disabling and life-shortening degenerative diseases.

To the health-promoting, disease-preventing diet

This is the diet based on unrefined starches, a diet high in fruit and vegetables, low in all refined foods. As faulty diet damages the tissues and eventually causes disease, so a healthy diet that eliminates the damaging animal products and the refined carbohydrates and fats will start to reverse the damage and help to prevent the chronic diseases from developing.

Therapeutic (healing) damage-reversing diet

This is the health-promoting diet taken a step further, aiming to eliminate all refined food and all animal

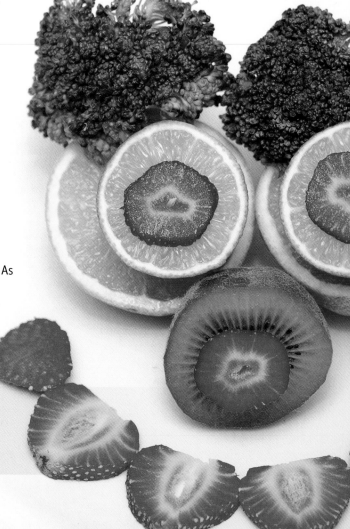

produce in order to get the full quota of nutrition from everything. A wide variety of whole plant foods, simply and appetisingly prepared, some of them fresh and raw, will give the body the optimum materials for damage reversal and healing. As wrong diet promotes the tissue damage that leads to disease, right diet promotes healing and damage reversal. As chronic degenerative diseases usually develop over many years, it may take a long time to reverse the changes, but small improvements can make big changes in symptoms, and one can expect to feel better in proportion to how much one can improve the diet and lifestyle.

Health reform is progressive, and sudden major changes are seldom necessary
Gradually replace refined foods with whole foods, and gradually phase out the animal products. This could take place over weeks, months or even a year, depending on how urgently improvement is needed, and how easily you adjust to the changes.

Start by adding more fruit and vegetables to your diet and reducing the amount of refined food.

Make a gradual changeover from white to whole-wheat bread and unrefined cereals.

Progress at your own pace – from meat-eater to semi-vegetarian (one who still eats

People already suffering with chronic degenerative problems like heart disease or diabetes will benefit very much from an improved diet and lifestyle, and should aim for the therapeutic diet. But it is very important to discuss any major diet or lifestyle changes that you plan to make with your medical advisors. This is especially important if you are on medication, because major lifestyle changes will affect (usually reduce) the amount of medication you need, and it is of course unwise or even dangerous to alter your medication without advice. There are still a few medical advisors who are sceptical about the ability of lifestyle changes to make a difference to chronic diseases, or of your ability to make and maintain those lifestyle changes, but most will welcome the prospect of improving your health and reducing your need for medical care.

some chicken and fish) to ovo-lacto vegetarian (one who eats plant foods plus dairy products and eggs). Once you are accustomed to eating a wide variety of natural, wholesome, unrefined plant foods and understand the principles of good nutrition, you can progress to a completely or almost completely plant-food (strict vegetarian or vegan) diet.

How strict do you need to be? That depends on what you want to achieve. It's the whole trend of your diet that is important, what you eat in the course of a week or month. Occasional items or even meals are not nearly so important as the whole trend.

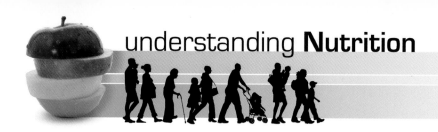
When urgent action is needed and you are really serious about it

Sometimes it's necessary to make changes quickly. Here is an easy regime which can be as flexible as you like – it can be done as suggested, over twelve days, but it could be eight days or even fewer. Or you could simply do the three-fruit-day part, which can be a very effective 'detox'. And, of course, it does depend on how your body responds to it.

Quick diet-change regime

Optional short fast – missing one or two meals and drinking plenty of clear fluids.

Stage 1: Three fruit days – meals composed of whatever fruits you enjoy, fresh, cooked, tinned, and so on, avoiding any strongly sweetened ones.

Stage 2: Three fruit-and-vegetable days – one or two fruit meals and a vegetable meal that consists of a variety of vegetables, some cooked, some raw.

Stage 3: Add whole-grain bread, brown rice or any other cereal products to your fruit and vegetable meals for the next three days.

Stage 4: For the next three days, add whatever you would like in the way of simple, whole-plant food proteins to complete the meals.

Stage 5: Long-term stage – continue as stage 4, or add whatever other things you want to include.

See chapter 8, **A total lifestyle plan for better health**, p. 106, for other lifestyle factors that will enhance the benefits of your change in diet.

Very important note

Some people expect a healthy diet to prevent them from ever getting ill. We can expect lifestyle changes to improve our health, postpone the onset of disease, and lengthen our lives, but there is no guarantee that they will prevent all disease. This is because there are factors beyond our control – the genetic makeup we have inherited from our parents for a start, and also environmental factors that we cannot control. However, genetic inheritance is not predestination: a healthy lifestyle will ensure that we make the very best of what we have.

Some frequently asked questions

Strict vegetarian or vegan?
All vegans are strict vegetarians, but not all strict vegetarians are vegans. Vegans avoid all exploitation of animals, so they avoid eating all foods of animal origin, including honey (a plant food concentrated and processed by bees). They are usually very healthy, but their primary motivation is not to be healthy so much as to avoid hurting or exploiting animals, which means that they try to avoid all animal products of every kind, including leather. Occasionally, people decide to be vegans and cut out all animal foods, without ensuring that all the plant foods they eat are whole and natural, and that is not healthy.

Strict vegetarians avoid eating all animal produce, but may not consider honey an animal produce, and they do not necessarily avoid non-food animal products.

Is a plant-food diet suitable for children?
Yes, but some thought and care is necessary at first. The plant-food diet has many advantages, but there are some possible problems, so here are some guidelines:

The principles are the same as for feeding all children – mother's milk only for the first six months if possible, then the gradual introduction of solid foods, keeping the baby's menu simple and being careful not to overload the diet with too many low-calorie, high-fibre fruits and vegetables. Soya baby milk can be used to mix the cereals and other foods.

Families with young children who are new to the plant-food diet will want more detailed information, for example, from the UK Vegan Society.

Benefits of whole-plant foods for children: there are many – more micronutrients, including iron, and vitamin C, which aids the absorption of iron, and many more phytochemicals, which boost the immune system. The avoidance of obesity is another major advantage.

Problems with whole-plant foods for children: there are a few, but they are easy to resolve. Babies and children need proportionately more calories than grownups, and this is true of adolescents too. On a whole-plant-food diet they could get too much fibre and not have room for the calories they need, and this is especially true of babies and toddlers. Another rather rare but potentially serious problem is vitamin B12 deficiency, especially if the mother is B12 deficient. (See note on B12 in the vitamin section on pages 50 and 51.)

Solution: more high-calorie, low-fibre foods. Rice is a relatively low-fibre cereal, and bananas are an excellent low-fibre, starchy food. Finely ground nuts, like almonds and cashews, and seeds, like sunflower and sesame, can be made into milks or creams and added to other foods to increase their calorie content. If there are B12 concerns,

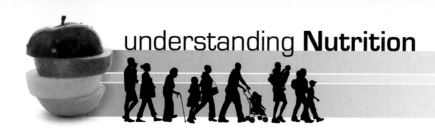
seek medical advice and get B12 supplements for the whole family if necessary.

What are 'empty calories'?

'Empty calories' is another term for junk food. These are the calories, or food energy units, that come from refined sugar, fats and starches. They include white sugar, vegetable oil, white flour, and all foods made mainly from them. Confectionery is mainly sugar; and soft drinks are sugared water. Cakes, biscuits and puddings are usually high in all three. Crisps and other savoury snacks are very high in fat, and also in salt. These foods provide very little more than fuel, because they have lost their vital nutrients and fibre. Having lost all or most of their minerals and vitamins, they do not contribute to health maintenance. Because they are so concentrated, they are not filling, and the temptation to overeat is hard to resist. They make a very major contribution to obesity and health problems of every kind.

Healthy and active people can usually cope with small amounts of junk food on an occasional basis, especially if they exercise vigorously to burn up the calories. If the junk food is a large part of the diet, there is a price to pay in present or future ill health, or both.

What about E-numbers and other additives?

E-numbers refer to food additives permitted in the EU. They include preservatives, colourings and stabilisers, and their use is a controversial subject. Some scientists reassure us that the additives are perfectly safe at the levels used, while others quote research that shows the opposite. The best plan is to avoid artificial additives as far as possible. This can be done by choosing a simple, natural diet using large amounts of fresh fruit and vegetables, some of them raw, and using simple, natural, homemade dishes rather than pre-packed ones. If this is our regular diet, we can be sure that our livers will be in the best possible condition to deal with whatever artificial additives and pollutants we may occasionally eat.

Is organic really better?

Organic food is produced without the use of artificial fertilisers and pesticides. It's still a controversial subject with conflicting evidence. It is important to understand that the enormous amount of evidence in favour of plant foods is not about organic plant foods. Plant foods, however they are grown, have health-promoting and healing properties.

For many people, a far more urgent question than how food is grown is how to get *enough* food. When a large proportion of the world's population goes hungry to bed, the organic farming question may seem largely irrelevant, a luxury to be adopted when everyone has enough to eat.

The organic lobby point out that organic methods are less damaging to the environment in both the short and the long term. Although many doubt that pesticide residues in food are dangerous, there is evidence of a higher incidence of many problems in farmers and others in close contact with pesticides in their work.

Organic varieties of certain foods taste better, but with others there is no difference, and for every research paper showing that their vitamin content is higher, there seems to be another that says it's not. Organic food also tends to be considerably more expensive. And, as it is often flown in from distant places, it may not be fresh.

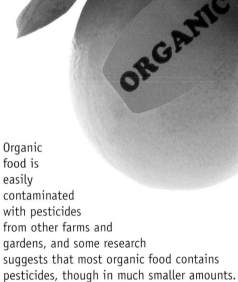

Organic food is easily contaminated with pesticides from other farms and gardens, and some research suggests that most organic food contains pesticides, though in much smaller amounts.

There's another reason to choose plant foods rather than animal foods. Pesticides are used in the production of animal feed. Animals concentrate the pesticides in their bodies and the food that animals produce for us to eat contains, weight for weight, more than ten times as much pesticide as plant foods do. Finally, the proportion of the different foods in the diet is probably more important than how they were grown: the more unrefined plant foods we eat, the greater our ability to deal with pollutants of all kinds.

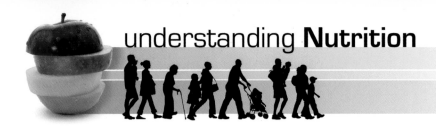

How safe are genetically modified foods?

Genetically modified food is another area where widely differing views are equally strongly held.

Plant breeders have been modifying crops by selective plant breeding for hundreds of years, but that process is too slow to meet the urgent need for more food. Others believe that genetic modification is inherently dangerous and wrong, and link it with increased risk of cancer and many other frightening prospects. Some say that only genetic modification can make plants resistant to disease and pesticides fast enough to feed the world's growing population.

There is persuasive evidence to suggest that the main danger of GM crops is to the environment, but there is less evidence of the harmful effects of actually eating the food. When we do not know the results of these types of interference with nature, it seems sensible to eat the simplest and most natural diet that is available. The ideal would be to grow our own food, and eat it when it's at its freshest and best. Failing that, we should eat a wide variety of the freshest and most natural food available and affordable, remembering that the important thing is the whole balance of our diets.

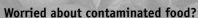

Worried about contaminated food?
Do the best that you can and eat with a thankful heart!

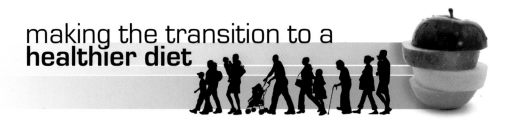
Is soya safe?

It depends upon whom you listen to. This is a controversial subject and the internet is full of websites on one side or the other. There are powerful interests involved, not least the soya-bean growers on one side and the dairy industry on the other.

The pro-soya lobby point to the many epidemiological studies that show an inverse relationship between soya consumption and reproductive cancer incidence. They also point to all the research that shows how soya helps lower cholesterol and so helps to prevent cardiovascular disease. They explain that the soya oestrogens that help to protect against hormone-related cancers also help protect against other hormonal problems, including painful periods and menopausal hot flushes. And they point out that millions of babies have been fed on soya milk formula since the 1930s with no evidence of harmful effects.

The anti-soya lobby have a list of frightening things to say: that the plant oestrogens in soya baby formula can feminise baby boys; that they also increase the incidence of breast cancer; that soya contributes to the development of serious thyroid problems, including cancer, and many more such dangers.

Who is right? There is a great deal of evidence in favour of soya, including impressive epidemiological studies. There is evidence on the other side, too, but much of it based on animal studies or small numbers of individual cases. This should also be balanced against the problems of dairy milk.

The jury may still be out on exactly how safe soya is and just who is at risk, but in the meantime there's little real evidence that small amounts of soya are harmful – say a cup of soya milk most days, and a serving of tofu or other soya-based product every few days.

Some people have gone over the top with soya, eating soya meat and dairy substitutes at almost every meal, and some have become ill, probably not so much due to the soya itself as to its excess. Neither tofu nor soya milk is a whole food and many soya products are very highly processed. The simple principle of keeping our diets simple, varied, based on unrefined starches, with plenty of fruit and vegetables and small amounts of beans, nuts and seeds should save us from most dietary problems, including those of soya.

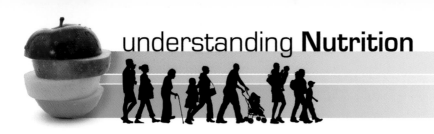

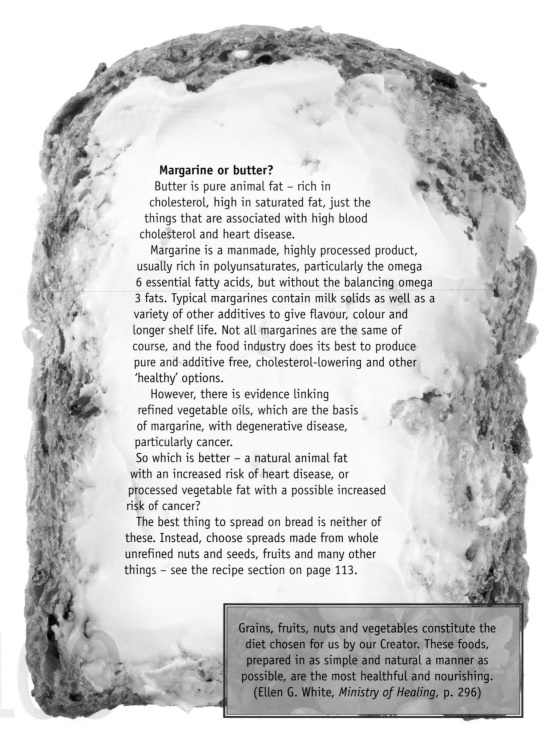

Margarine or butter?

Butter is pure animal fat – rich in cholesterol, high in saturated fat, just the things that are associated with high blood cholesterol and heart disease.

Margarine is a manmade, highly processed product, usually rich in polyunsaturates, particularly the omega 6 essential fatty acids, but without the balancing omega 3 fats. Typical margarines contain milk solids as well as a variety of other additives to give flavour, colour and longer shelf life. Not all margarines are the same of course, and the food industry does its best to produce pure and additive free, cholesterol-lowering and other 'healthy' options.

However, there is evidence linking refined vegetable oils, which are the basis of margarine, with degenerative disease, particularly cancer.

So which is better – a natural animal fat with an increased risk of heart disease, or processed vegetable fat with a possible increased risk of cancer?

The best thing to spread on bread is neither of these. Instead, choose spreads made from whole unrefined nuts and seeds, fruits and many other things – see the recipe section on page 113.

> Grains, fruits, nuts and vegetables constitute the diet chosen for us by our Creator. These foods, prepared in as simple and natural a manner as possible, are the most healthful and nourishing.
> (Ellen G. White, *Ministry of Healing*, p. 296)

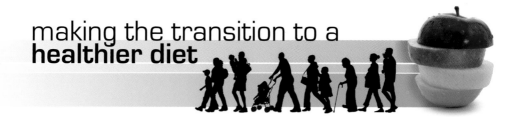

making the transition to a healthier diet

What about fasting?

Fasting gives the digestive organs and liver a rest, or 'detox'. It also helps one to develop self-control, which is no bad thing when struggling with overweight or other health problems.

A short fast can be very helpful when one is stressed, tired, or feeling unwell for a variety of reasons. A fast could be as simple as missing a meal, or it could be a whole day with only water and herb teas. Another way of giving the digestive system and liver a rest is to eat only fruit for one or two days. Anyone who is underweight should be careful about fasts, but people who struggle with their weight might benefit from short fasts on a regular basis.

products, plus a generous supply of high-water-content vegetables or fruit, and a smaller amount of high-protein food. Food is easier to digest and it is easier not to overeat if there is less variety at any one meal, but

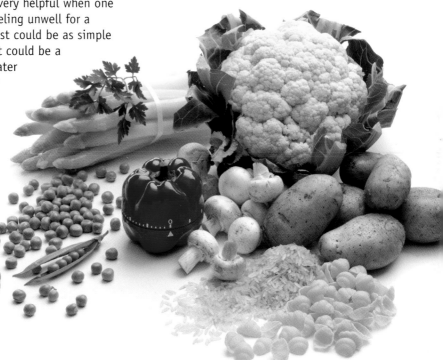

Practical advice about eating for health

Choosing a variety of whole, unrefined plant foods ensures an adequate supply of all the essential nutrients (with the possible exception of vitamin B12, and in certain circumstances vitamin D; see chapter on vitamins). A varied diet protects against possible deficiencies, and also the boredom and food cravings that cause so many diets to fail. The basis of a healthy diet should be unrefined starches – rice, potatoes, whole-wheat bread and pasta, and other cereal

it is important to have a wide variety of food from day to day.

There are other very important factors in our choice of foods – the climate, the season, our occupation, age and life situation. Fewer calories are needed in hot weather; more are needed by manual workers. Growing children need proportionally more calories, as do pregnant and nursing mothers; the elderly need fewer. Then there are individual health factors – illnesses, food intolerances and allergies.

Economic considerations and food availability are the most important factors in food choice for many. Whatever the situation, they must do the best they can. In limited situations, they should choose the widest variety of the most nutritious food available.

Guide to planning meals

The healthiest diets worldwide are those based on unrefined starches. Add to the starch plenty of fruit and vegetables and some of the more concentrated foods – beans, lentils, nuts and seeds. Prepare them simply without unnecessary added fat, sugar or spices, and enjoy them!

Deciding when to eat

Meal timing is important because the digestive system works best on a regular schedule. An average meal needs over four hours in the stomach. Mealtimes at least five hours apart give the stomach time for rest and recovery. Ideally, the evening meal should be the lightest and it should end several hours before bedtime, so the stomach can rest while we sleep. This will also ensure deeper and more refreshing sleep and a good appetite for breakfast.

Choosing what to eat

Asterisks indicate recipes in this book. See recipe section, pages 113-133.

Breakfast should be simple, quick and easy to prepare, but substantial – a main meal, in fact. Many people choose a fruit and grain meal – say, fruit, cereal and toast.

Cereals: if you want packet cereals, choose those made from whole-wheat and other grains, without added sugar. You can make hot breakfast cereals from a variety of flaked whole grains, as well as from porridge oats.

Alternatives to dairy milk: fresh or cooked fruit, fruit juice or smoothie,* soya or nut milk.* Sweetenings and other toppings: use raisins or chopped dates instead of sugar. Granola* and chopped nuts make delicious crunchy toppings for hot cereals.

Bread: choose whole varieties of bread and crisp-bread and vary them from day to day.

Spreads: choose ones that contain their full spectrum of nutrition – whole nut butters,* tahini, avocado (an excellent substitute for cream cheese), mashed banana. Delicious 'jams'* can be very easily made from dried fruits, cooked and mashed or blended.

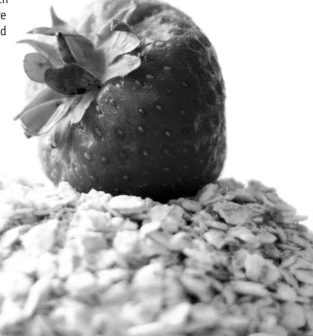

making the transition to a
healthier diet

Fruit: include several kinds, fresh, cooked or dried, some to eat with cereal, some on bread, some on their own.
Savoury breakfasts* are good too.

The midday meal – this should ideally
be the other main meal. A simple, light dessert* is optional for either meal.

A 'cooked lunch'
The filling, starchy part: choice of steamed or baked potato, brown rice, brown pasta, maize, and so on.

The vegetables: several kinds and colours, some cooked, some raw.

The high protein food: choose a small amount of these – the pulse, nut and seed group. They could just be some interesting items added to rice or pasta, or they could be separate dishes, for example, a nut roast* or bean stew.**

Sauces and dressings are important as food needs to be appetising, but they should be chosen carefully, because few of the ones in the shops are really healthy.

A 'light lunch'
Starchy part: bread or crisp-bread.

Vegetables: soup or a salad, or both.

Protein: can be in a spread form such as hummus or nut butter, or it could be lentil or bean soup.*

The evening meal – it is best to have
the lightest meal in the evening if it's possible. This is because the food you eat in the evening tends to be stored as fat, and large evening meals keep the stomach working well into the night when it needs to rest.

Bread and spread with fruit, or bread and spread with a soup or salad, or simply fruit – each is a good evening menu.

Drinks with meals?
Drinking large amounts of fluids with meals, especially if they are cold, dilutes the digestive juices and slows digestion down. The best time for drinking is between meals, and it's a good plan to keep drinks with meals to a minimum. If you have plenty of water between meals and plenty of vegetables and fruits on the menu, there will be less need to drink with meals.

What about skipping meals?
If you are not underweight, by all means occasionally skip a meal, and give your digestive system a rest. But it's a big mistake

103

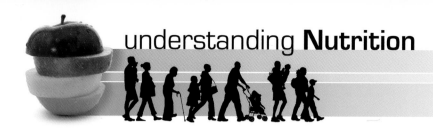
to miss breakfast on a regular basis. When stressed, overworked, or unwell in general, your missing one or two evening meals can be very helpful, so much so, that many people decide they are better on a two-meal plan.

Fruits and vegetables at the same meal?

Some people find them difficult to digest together. Others simply find it's a useful policy to keep them separate if there are health or weight problems, as it keeps things simple and it's easier not to overeat.

What are the rules for food combining?

The most important rule is **eat a wide variety of whole unrefined plant foods, but keep the individual meals simple and do not overeat.**

There used to be a very popular food combining theory based on the fact that the amino acids in plant proteins come in slightly different combinations from those in animal proteins. According to this theory, the 'complete' animal combination of amino acids must be provided at every meal. For example, wheat could be complemented with beans, which was nice for everyone who liked beans on toast. However there is no need to match the amino acids at every meal. The amino acids do not all need to be supplied at the same time, and, provided we eat a variety of different

vegetable proteins from day to day, there will be plenty.

Another older and more complicated food combining theory is that protein and starch should not be eaten together. This means that beans on toast are out, along with the corn and beans of Mexico, the rice and dahl of India, Chinese rice and tofu and most kinds of sandwiches. There is no scientific evidence for this theory, which is as well, because it can make eating with other people very difficult, and it

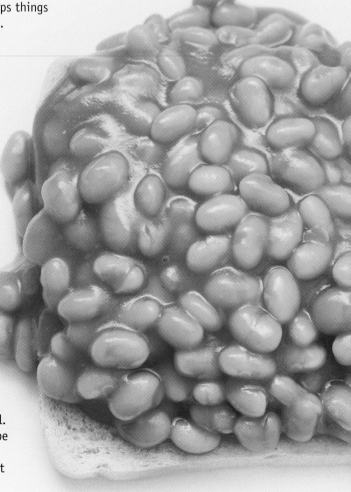

is impossible to follow anyway, because whole plant foods are not made of single nutrients. Grains contain protein, beans and lentils contain starch, and even fruits and vegetables contain protein, though in small amounts. Some people claim to have been helped very much by carefully following this regime, but the benefit is due to eating simpler and more natural foods, not to the way they are combined.

> These are ideals to aim for. Do not be discouraged if it's impossible to meet the ideal standard, because of shift-work, family commitments and other factors. Do the best you can, and remember that health reform is progressive, and be ready to make improvements when you are able.

What if you cannot choose the menu?

If you do not have any say about what happens in the kitchen, you can still make choices that will improve your diet and health.

First, *do not add sugar* and avoid sugar-rich foods. Get your own supplies of other foods, such as fruits or nuts to take their place if possible.

Be very careful about fats. Cultivate a taste for less. Remember, fats come on bread as butter and margarine, are plentiful in fried food, but are also present in large amounts in many gravies, sauces and made-up dishes such as stews and casseroles. Pastry is by weight at least one third fat, and cakes, biscuits and ice-cream are often as rich in fats as they are in sugar. Be careful about cheese – standard hard cheeses like cheddar are over 50% fat. *Eat bigger helpings of the vegetables and salads, and smaller helpings of the high-fat foods,* avoiding the richest altogether. This will save you many empty calories. And do not forget that exercise can go a long way towards making up for a less than ideal diet.

How strict does one have to be?

This is something you need to decide for yourself, according to how good your general health is, whether you need to lose (or even gain) weight, what your social circumstances are and so on. Occasional deviations from your healthy eating plan may be unavoidable, but regular indulgence in junk food makes it more difficult to develop a taste for the better things. As time passes, if you manage to avoid the dangerous fattening foods, you will find that *you develop a taste for the healthy food*. As you start to feel better on the new regime, you are even more motivated to continue it. Some people find that it is best to be total abstainers from rich cakes and puddings, as they may set off cravings that are hard to control. Others can take them or leave them and have no problems with eating them occasionally on social occasions. The problem is when one feels the need to eat junk food to reward oneself for abstaining from it! That is likely to lead to the slippery slope of failure.

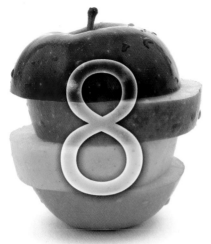

Diet isn't everything

A total lifestyle plan for better health

NEW START is a rehabilitation programme developed by doctors in the late 1970s at Weimar Institute in California. Thousands have been through the programme, and it has been particularly successful in helping people with high blood pressure, high blood cholesterol, coronary heart disease, diabetes and weight problems. NEW START is an acronym for eight natural remedies – **Nutrition, Exercise, Water, Sunlight, Temperance, Air, Rest, Trust in Divine Power** – on which the programme is based.

Putting the NEW START programme into practice:

Nutrition recap – **The therapeutic diet principles behind the New Start Plan**

1) The 'Revolutionary' Eating Plan:
 Big breakfast, moderate lunch, small supper, because the food we eat in the morning provides energy for the day, but much food eaten in the evening is stored as fat.

2) The Totally Nutritious Plant Food Plan
 All the food is whole and unrefined, with all its vitamins, minerals, and fibre intact, all of which are needed for staying well or getting better.

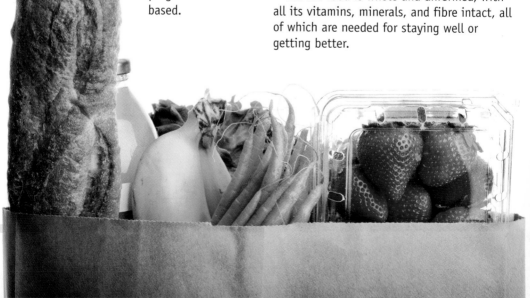

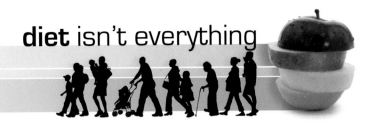

diet isn't everything

3) The Raw-food Emphasis Plan

Something raw at every meal – because fresh, raw food is very rich in vitamins, minerals and other health-promoting substances.

4) The Varied-diet Plan

A wide variety of foods from day to day, but not too many different things at any one meal.

Exercise: Regular enjoyable daily exercise

– up to one hour or more according to tolerance – preferably in the fresh air and sunlight, because exercise is as important as diet in fighting disease.

Water: good hydration is vital for health

and is easy if you start with a large drink of water (hot or cold) on waking (at least half an hour before breakfast), then drink mid-morning, mid-afternoon and mid-evening. (Exact amounts depend on the individual: drink enough to keep the urine pale and clear).

Sunlight: Sunlight in moderation is

therapeutic. It helps to reduce stress and lower cholesterol and is essential for the production of vitamin D in our bodies. A light tan protects the skin from sun damage, as does a plant-food diet.

Temperance: This means avoiding

poisons – caffeine, alcohol, 'recreational drugs'; unnecessary medications and even highly seasoned foods and condiments which all place added burdens on the body. It also means avoiding all extremes in the practice of health principles as well as in diet.

Air: Clean air indoors and out as far as

possible, with well-ventilated rooms and outdoor exercise in the most natural environment available.

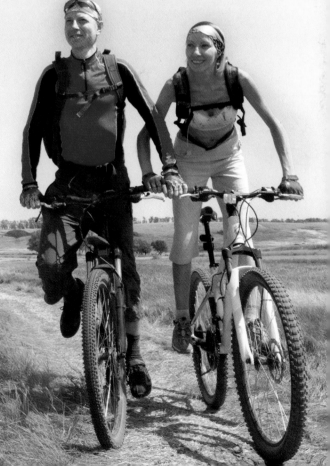

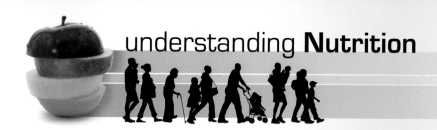

Rest: The aim is adequate night-time rest, which for most people is between seven and eight hours of sleep (NB: early nights are much more refreshing than late mornings). Weekly rest days and regular holidays are also vital for physical and mental health. Our stomachs need rest too. Eating between meals or eating too many meals keeps our stomachs constantly at work. Three meals a day is as much as most stomachs can deal with on a regular basis, and many people are better with two.

Reminder

All who have serious health problems, particularly if they are on regular medication, should consult their medical advisor before starting to make major lifestyle changes.

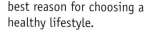

Trust in Divine Power:

The right mental attitude is the most powerful of all the healing factors. Trust in divine power has a lot to do with a healthy mental attitude that enhances our health and enables our bodies to make the best use of the food we eat. It provides a basis for optimism, cheerfulness, thankfulness and interest in and concern for others. There is plenty of research evidence to show that these attitudes are associated with longer, healthier lives, as well as better digestion. It also provides the best and most lasting motivation for the lifestyle changes that most of us need to make when we are faced with the prospect of ill health. The knowledge that the Creator who designed our amazingly complex and wonderful bodies also designed the vast variety of delicious and beautiful plant foods for us to enjoy is the best reason for choosing a healthy lifestyle.

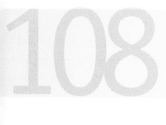

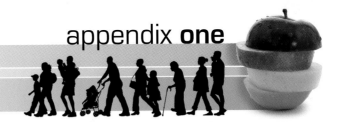
Appendix 1

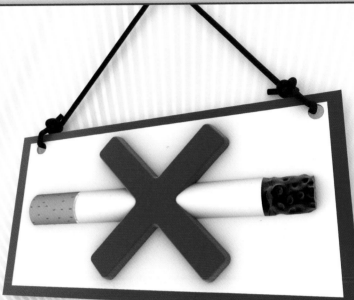

Seventh-day Adventists and longer, healthier lives

There is a much-studied group of people who seem to have made a successful investment in their health – the Seventh-day Adventists. Over 300 peer-reviewed scientific papers testify to the Adventist health advantage. When all things are considered, as far as the UK and USA are concerned, Adventist men and women, *who follow the Adventist lifestyle*, can expect an extra ten and eight years respectively, and, even more interestingly, these extra years come with the bonus of less disability too. The extra years are healthy years.

What is the Adventist secret? Adventists believe in stewardship of their health – their bodies belong to God and they have a duty to keep them as healthy as possible. That is why smoking tobacco and drinking alcohol are not part of the lifestyle, and this gives them a head start where life-shortening diseases are concerned, and explains their lower overall incidence of heart disease, stroke and cancer. Some of the most interesting information is from the Loma Linda Adventist Health Study, which has tracked the health of many thousands of Adventists for over thirty years. This is important research, because although most Adventists have a similar stand on alcohol, tobacco, the weekly rest day and the need to eat healthily, there is quite a range of interpretations as to what healthy eating means. Researchers have been able to compare the health and longevity of meat-eating, ovo-lacto-vegetarian and strict-vegetarian Adventists, and have found some interesting results.

All the groups had an advantage over the general population with regard to heart disease, stroke and cancer.

- The meat-eating group had the smallest advantage (about 50% less disease).
- The strict-vegetarian or vegan group had the biggest advantage (about 85% less).
- The ovo-lacto vegetarians were in between (with about 65% less).
- The health advantage was greater the earlier in life the lifestyle was started.

How do the Adventists come to have this health emphasis?

It was back in the middle of the nineteenth century that Adventist health pioneer Ellen G. White called the Church's attention to the Bible's emphasis on stewardship of health, and the Creator's original plan for a vegetarian diet and a healthy, active, outdoor lifestyle. While still in her early twenties, she pointed out the health hazards of tea, coffee and tobacco, and soon she was recommending hydrotherapy. This was a great advance in those times of medical ignorance, when dangerous drugs were in common use for minor ailments, and tobacco smoking was prescribed for lung diseases. From the middle of the 1860s she was actively involved in speaking and writing about the health benefits of a simple, wholesome vegetarian diet, active exercise, water drinking and the avoidance of poisons, including the drugs prescribed by many physicians as well as alcohol, tobacco and caffeine. She also encouraged the establishing of sanitariums where doctors would use only natural methods. Her teaching on both the laws of health and the remedies for disease are summed up as

> **'Pure air, sunlight, abstemiousness, rest, exercise, proper diet, the use of water, trust in divine power, these are the true remedies.'** (*Ministry of Healing*, page 127.)

Adventists have a priceless heritage in these teachings. Each individual has the opportunity to choose a well-proven healthier lifestyle. It's a secret they have kept for too long and one that everyone can choose to benefit from.

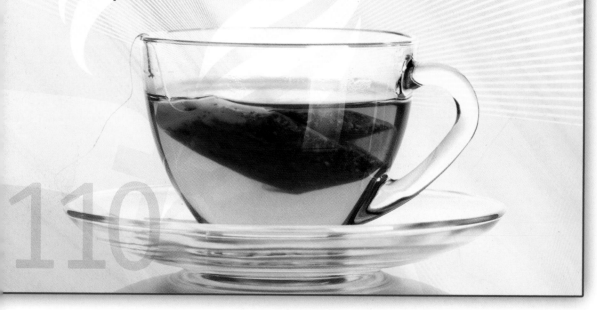

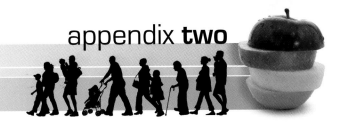

Appendix 2

Taking charge of your digestive system

Digestive problems have many causes, but the most common ones have to do with unhealthy diet and eating habits, lack of exercise, negative mental attitudes and the use of harmful substances. Everyone is different, and what upsets one may not upset another, but healthy diet and eating habits, exercise, positive mental attitudes and the avoidance of harmful substances will work wonders for most digestive problems. So, if your digestive system plays up from time to time, go through these checklists and see what you can do. The solution is in your hands and on your plate.

Irritants that can cause trouble

1. Hot pepper (black or red), spices (including ginger, cinnamon, cloves, nutmeg), mustard.
2. Vinegar and things made with vinegar (pickles, salad dressings, ketchup, and so on).
3. Foods made with baking soda or baking powder.
4. Fatty or oily foods (fried foods, pastry, sausages, fatty meats).
5. Sugar and rich sugary foods.
6. Tea, coffee and chocolate.
7. Alcohol.
8. Smoking.
9. Aspirin and other anti-inflammatory medicines (for example iboprofen).
10. Worry and other negative mental attitudes.

Eating habits that spell danger

1. Eating too often, especially between meals.
2. Eating too much.
3. Eating late at night.
4. Drinking large amounts of fluids with meals.
5. Eating when anxious, upset or very tired.

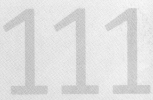

111

Eating habits that help to heal

1. Eating at regular mealtimes, with at least five hours between the end of one meal and the start of the next, and several hours between the last meal and bedtime.

2. Eating mainly at breakfast and lunch, keeping the evening meal small and light – or even omitting it for a while, or regularly.

3. Simple but varied meals – a small variety of food at any one meal, but a wide variety from day to day.

4. Eating mainly whole-plant foods (minimum of sugar, fat and other refined foods).

5. Drinking mainly water, with plenty *between* meals, and drinking little of anything at all *with* meals.

6. Eating calmly, cheerfully, and with a thankful heart.

Other habits that promote healthy digestion

1. exercise – a short, brisk walk after meals promotes the action of the stomach, getting digestion off to a good start, while strenuous exercise soon after meals has the opposite effect.

Regular vigorous exercise has a beneficial effect on all the organs of the body, including the whole of the digestive tract.

2. rest – all systems work better with regular and adequate periods of rest. To give the digestive system a rest, avoid eating between meals, and overeating. If necessary, miss an evening meal or even several evening meals. Remember that rest for the whole person includes not only regular and adequate sleep, but also rest days and holidays.

3. positive thinking – stress, worry and negative thinking are important factors in many digestive problems, and replacing these with more positive reactions and attitudes helps to heal and restore.

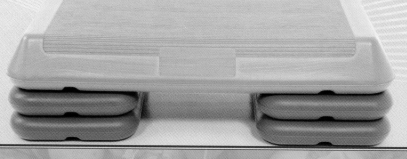

Important note:
Always seek medical advice for persistent new symptoms or when serious problems are suspected. These health principles are complementary and can be expected to enhance the effect of medical treatment if it is necessary. When in doubt, seek professional advice.

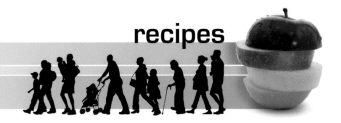

recipes to help with starting the whole-plant-food diet

equipment

It is perfectly possible to eat a very healthy plant-food diet using very basic equipment, however a blender with a coffee mill attachment is a good investment, and is strongly recommended. It saves a lot of time and greatly increases the range of things that can be made at home.

note re oil, salt and seasonings

Below is a small selection of recipes to help with the transition from the typical Western diet, with its strong emphasis on dairy and other animal produce, to an interesting, health-promoting, whole-plant-food diet, or, if necessary, to a therapeutic diet. Some recipes use a little olive oil, but it can be omitted if desired. As most people eat too much salt, we recommend that avoiding the high salt processed foods, eating plenty of fruit, not adding salt to cooked cereals or sweet things, and cultivating a taste for less salt in savoury things. These recipes are flexible and basic, so as far as salt and other seasonings are concerned, the advice is 'according to your taste'. The principle is, go easy on the salt and other seasonings, remembering that herbs are helpful, but strong spices are not.

measurements

Standard cup and spoon measurements are used in these recipes. Cups are easier and quicker than scales, and are especially useful for plant food cookery, which tends to be more flexible, and doesn't often need such exact measurements.

1 cup = 250ml = one standard tea cup
½ cup = 125ml
¼ cup = 62.5ml = (roughly) 4tbs
1 standard tablespoon (1tbs) = 15ml = ½ an old fashioned household tablespoon
1 standard teaspoon (1tsp) = 5ml = 1 old fashioned teaspoon

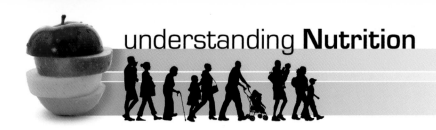

breakfast recipes

cooked cereals

Porridge oats are the quickest and easiest cereal to cook, but there are other types of cereal flakes that make good breakfasts for cold mornings.

For two people, use 1 cup oat or other cereal flakes, 2½-3 cups water, depending on how thick you want it to be. Bring it to the boil, stirring occasionally, then turn down and simmer until it's cooked. Porridge oats take about 5 minutes, rice and millet flakes 10 minutes, barley and rye flakes 20 minutes – less time if you pour boiling water over the flakes half an hour earlier.

muesli

The original muesli, invented by Dr Bircher Benner more than a hundred years ago, was thoroughly soaked overnight to ensure that the grains were digestible, and the largest ingredient was the fresh fruit that was added in the morning.

Here is a variation on muesli:

Cool and creamy oatmeal
2 cups porridge oats
2 cups orange juice
½ cup chopped nuts
4-6 cups fresh fruit
Combine the first 3 ingredients and refrigerate over night. Just before serving, mix in the prepared fresh fruit, e.g. grated apples, chopped pears, peaches, apricots, berries.

granola

Granola is delicious and easy to make and keeps well in an airtight box or tin. It can be used as a crunchy topping to porridge or stewed fruit, and is also useful for making piecrusts. The recipes below are very flexible. Granola is made from a mixture of cereal flakes (usually oats), with nuts and seeds and sweetening which can be honey, malt, fruit juice concentrate, mashed bananas, dates or apple sauce. The proportions can be varied. It should only be moist enough to be crumbly – big lumps take longer to cook. If you want to include raisins or other dried fruit, add them after cooking or they will get hard. Add a tiny bit of salt if you want to, but it isn't really necessary for most tastes. A little oil will make for a crispier granola, but also one that will burn more easily. Cook slowly, say at 150°C, checking and stirring occasionally.

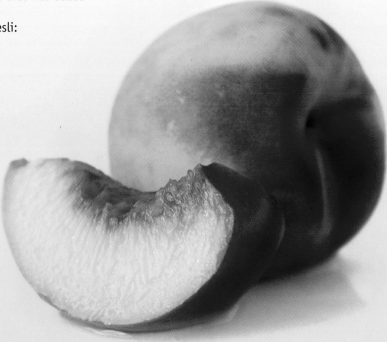

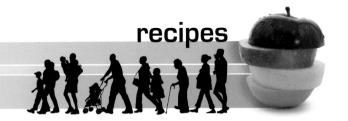

Recipe 1

4 cups porridge oats
½ cup desiccated coconut
½ cup pumpkin or sunflower seeds
¾ cup chopped nuts, blended with just enough water to cover them
¼ teaspoon vanilla
4 tablespoons apple juice concentrate or honey

Mix together thoroughly and spread on 2 baking trays. Bake in a slow oven until golden brown and crunchy. Check and stir occasionally while baking.

Recipe 2

1 cup pitted dates, softened in enough hot water to cover
2 ripe bananas
8 cups rolled oats
1 cup chopped nuts
1 cup desiccated coconut
1 cup sunflower seeds
½ tsp vanilla essence

Blend the first 2 ingredients until smooth, then mix thoroughly with everything else. Spread about ½ inch thick on trays and bake in a cool oven for about 1½ hours, stirring occasionally.

'milks' and other things to eat with cereals

Cashew 'milk' or cream

Blend 1 cup cashews in 1 cup water until very smooth – about 1 minute, less if you cook them (in just enough water to cover) for a few minutes first. Blend briefly with 3-4 cups of water for milk, proportionately less for cream. You can use other nuts, such as Brazil nuts or almonds, but cashews are the creamiest.

Cashew rice or oat 'milk'

½ cup cashews
½ cup cooked brown rice or cooked oats (left over porridge)

Add enough water to cover, and blend until smooth. Stir before serving.

Sesame 'milk'

Blend light tahini together with 4 or 5 parts of water. Add more water as desired. This is rather an acquired taste, but those who do acquire the taste love it. It's a rich source of calcium.

Sweetening 'milk'

Those who want to can sweeten their milk with a little apple juice concentrate, honey or malt, or blend in a couple of softened dates. A little vanilla or almond essence can be added too.

Fruit whip
Blend together 1 cup pineapple or orange juice with a banana and use as milk with breakfast cereal.

nut butters

Use either raw or roasted nuts. Cashews, peanuts, almonds and hazelnuts make particularly good butters if they are roasted first. Walnuts, pecans and Brazil nuts make good butters just as they are.

To make a small amount of nut butter, grind ¼ cup nuts to a fine consistency in a coffee grinder. If necessary mix it with a little water or oil to make it spreadable. Adding water gives an excellent creamy spread that keeps for a few days in the fridge. If you use oil rather than water, it will keep for much longer.

To make nut butter in a blender, grind up one cupful of nuts at a time, and add water or oil as needed.

You can make your own tahini with toasted sesame seeds in a coffee grinder in the same way as nut butters and you can make sunflower and pumpkin seed butters in the same way.

'jams'

Dried fruit jams
You can use one or more kinds of dried fruit. For soft, 'ready to eat' dried fruit, you can just pour boiling water over it and let it soak until it's soft, then mash or blend.

For more chewy dried fruit, you may like to cook it as well. Soak first, for an hour or more, then cook gently until it's fairly soft, then mash or blend.

Date spread
1 cup chopped dates with enough hot water to cover
　　Just soak until soft and stir.

Variations: use orange juice instead of water; stir in ¼ tsp ground aniseed or cardamom.

Apricot and pear spread
Cook a mixture of dried apricots and dried pears in enough water to cover them. Mash or blend, depending how smooth you like it to be.

Fresh or frozen fruit jams
Use any sort of fresh or frozen fruit you like. Cook briefly and use chopped dates or raisins to sweeten and thicken: Use 1 cup dates to 1-2 cups fruit, depending on how sweet the fruit is.

Blackcurrant spread
1 cup fresh blackcurrants (use slightly more if using frozen fruit)
1 cup chopped dates
Water – just enough to cover the dates.
Cook the dates in the water for a few minutes, then add the fresh or frozen fruit, bring it to the boil, stir well, then leave it to cool. It will thicken as it cools. Add more water for a thinner spread.

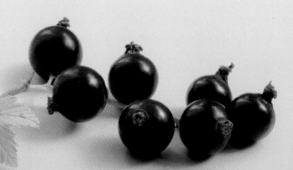

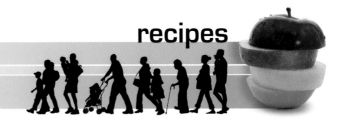

savoury dishes for main meals

basic savoury nut recipe

(for four)

1 cup nuts
2 cups breadcrumbs
1 large onion
1 stick celery
½ cup water
1 tbs yeast extract
1 tbs mixed herbs

Make the breadcrumbs and then grind the nuts in the blender. Next blend the onion, celery, yeast extract and ½ cup water together. Now mix everything together and stir in the herbs. The mixture should be moist but firm. Add more water if it is too dry.

For a **nut roast**, put the mixture in a well-greased loaf tin and cook in a moderate oven for an hour or more, until it is fairly firm. Or put it in a shallow tin or casserole dish, and it will bake more quickly.

For **burgers or patties**, form into balls, then place on oiled tray, flatten into desired shape and bake in a moderate oven. These will cook much more quickly than the roast – in half an hour or less. Turn them once during cooking for a flatter shape.

For **pâté**, bake in the oven until just firm. Cool and spread on bread.

For **pie**, make a whole wheat-oat pie shell, put a layer of steamed or sautéed onion, then cover with nut roast mixture and bake.

For **stuffed marrow**, first cut the marrow in half longways, scoop out the seeds, half cook it in the oven, a steamer or microwave oven. Then fill the marrow with the nut mixture, and bake in a moderate oven until the marrow is fully cooked and the stuffing is firm and starting to brown.

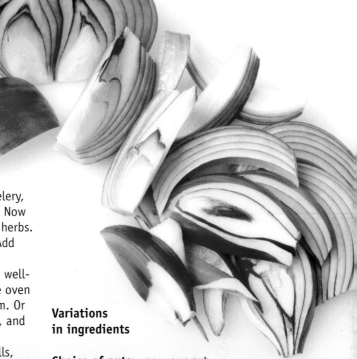

Variations in ingredients

Choice of nuts: vary your nut roasts by choosing different varieties of nuts, different herbs, different vegetables and even different kinds of bread or other starches. Peanuts are the cheapest nuts and mix well with most other nuts when used half and half. You can also use sunflower seeds to replace half or all of the nuts. For a start try walnuts with peanuts, hazelnuts with sunflower seeds.

Choice of vegetables: add a carrot instead of or as well as the onion or celery.

Choice of herbs and other flavourings: the possibilities are endless.

Choice of starchy basis: instead of

117

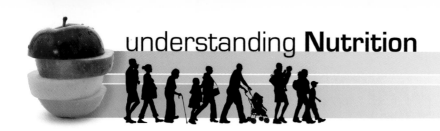
breadcrumbs you can use mashed potato, cooked rice or cooked millet, reducing the water for blending the onion by half. Replacing some of the breadcrumbs, say a quarter to a third, with rye bread adds a rich flavour. The mixture should be moist but firm. If it is too moist, add a handful of porridge oats to absorb the excess moisture.

This is quite a rich nut roast. If you feel it is too rich, simply alter the proportions, reducing the amount of nuts, and/or increasing the amount of breadcrumbs or other starch. It's the sort of recipe that really cannot easily go wrong.

Menu planning: nut roast is for eating as part of a main course, with plenty of salad, cooked vegetables, and unrefined starch in the form of potatoes, rice, etc. It is not supposed to be eaten by the plateful on its own. Nut pâté on bread makes a good meal with vegetable soup and salad.

chestnuts with brown lentils

Use Puy lentils, or 'green' lentils (which are brownish-green before cooking). These lentils do not need to be soaked, but take up to an hour to cook.

1 medium onion, chopped
1-2 cloves garlic, crushed
1 stick celery, chopped
1 tbs olive oil, plus 1 tbs water
1 cup lentils
1 tin or pack ready to eat chestnuts (240g)
Yeast extract, or other seasoning to taste

Sauté the onion and garlic in the oil and water. Add the lentils and enough boiling water to cover them. Cover the pan and simmer gently, adding more water later if necessary, until the lentils are soft. Add the chestnuts and the yeast extract or other seasoning, heat through and serve.

Variations: oil free – omit the sautéing stage, and simply cook everything together from the start.

No chestnuts available? Just make it a vegetable and lentil stew with carrots, red or yellow peppers, etc.

118

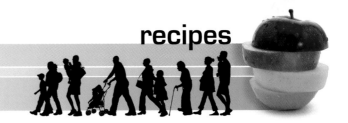

some bean recipes

bean and vegetable stew

Beans need to be soaked overnight and then cooked for an hour or more. It saves time to cook a quantity and freeze them until you need them. If using ready cooked or tinned beans, you can either sauté the chopped onion and celery and garlic in a little olive oil or water, before adding the other vegetables and the beans, or you can omit the oil and just put everything in the pan together. For a winter stew, add sliced carrots, chunks of potato, swede, parsnip, your choice of herbs and other seasonings and the ready cooked beans, plus enough water to keep it from burning. Cook gently until the vegetables are done. For a Provençal flavour use courgettes, peppers, aubergines, tomatoes, ready cooked beans and flavouring. If you would like to thicken the stew, stir in 1 tbs flour or cornflour, mixed to a smooth paste with ½ cup of water, and stir gently for a few minutes until it thickens.

butter bean casserole

1 tin butter beans (1½ cups cooked beans)
1 cupful *creamy cashew sauce* (see page 125)
   Pour the sauce over the beans in a small ovenproof dish and bake in a moderate oven until the top begins to brown.

bean burgers

Do it all in a food processor if you have one, otherwise mash beans and chop onion finely.
1 cup beans
1 medium onion
1 cup mashed potato (or breadcrumbs)
Choice of flavourings:
   1) Tomato purée, oregano, garlic, chopped olives (½ cup)
   2) Yeast extract, mixed herbs
   3) Coriander, cumin and garlic
   Mix everything together, adding some soya milk or water if necessary. Form into patties or burgers and place on an oiled or non-stick baking tray. Bake for about half an hour in a moderate oven until golden brown. Serve them in buns with sliced onion, and catsup or sliced tomato, or for dinner with cooked vegetables and gravy or tomato sauce.

bean spreads

You can give the blender a rest and simply mash the cooked or tinned beans with a little water or soya milk. There are endless variations to be made, so just use your imagination and whatever you can find in your cupboard. Here are two to start you off.
Mediterranean: add olive oil, tomato purée, herbs – basil and/or oregano, chopped olives.
English Special: mash the beans with a generous amount of Marmite. Mix well. Eat on toast.

119

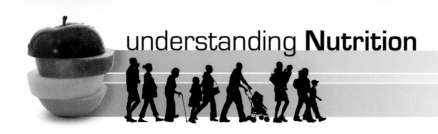

some 'cheeze' ideas

Do not think of 'cheese substitute' but of 'interesting vege spreads.' When you get used to them, you may well prefer them, especially as they are lighter and easier to digest than dairy cheese. Use them in sandwiches, on toast or pizza.

country life cashew pimento cheeze

Blend until smooth:

1 cup water
¾ cup cashew nuts or sunflower seeds
2 tbs sesame seeds or tahini
⅔ cup rolled oats
3 tbs yeast flakes
1 small onion
1 level tsp herb salt
1 clove garlic
2 tbs lemon juice, or to taste
½ cup tinned or fresh pimentos (sweet peppers)
⅛ tsp dill seed (optional)

This can be used as it is in lasagne, for pizza topping, or 'cheeze' on toast. It can be added to a white sauce for cauliflower 'cheeze'.

To make a spread for sandwiches, cook it until it thickens, stirring all the time.

To make into a brick for slicing, mix 4 tbs agar flakes in 1½ cups water and boil until flakes are dissolved. Use the above recipe, but substitute the 1½ cups agar mixture for the 1 cup water. Blend until creamy then pour into a mould and chill.

quick cheeze sauce

1 cup cashew pieces cooked for a few minutes in 1 cup water
3 tbs yeast flakes
1 tsp salt
¼ cup fresh onion
1 clove garlic
½ cup pimento or sweet pepper, cooked or chopped (leave out for white 'cheeze')
2 tbs lemon juice

Blend until very creamy. Use as it is for pizza, lasagne or 'cheeze' on toast. Cook to use as a spread.

lighter cheeze sauce

To make a lighter cheeze sauce, for cauliflower 'cheeze', etc.: mix one part of cheeze sauce with one or two parts of white sauce (made with 2 tbs flour to one cup of soya or other milk).

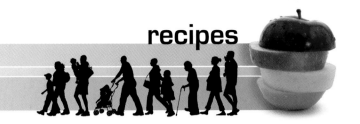

some tofu recipes

scrambled tofu

Forget scrambled eggs – it's not the same at all – but scrambled tofu can be very good in its own right. Serve it on toast with some cooked or raw tomato, and anything else you would like to eat with it.

1 large onion, chopped
1 stick celery, chopped
2 tbs olive oil with 1 tbs water (oil-free version – use 3 tbs soya milk)
1 250g block tofu
1 clove garlic, crushed
1 tbs yeast flakes
1 tsp herb salt
¼ tsp turmeric
Soya milk

Sauté the first 3 ingredients together until soft and transparent, then mash or blend before adding the crumbled tofu and seasonings. If you would like it to be more creamy, add soya milk until it is the desired consistency. Mix well and heat through.

tofu cottage cheeze

1 250g pack of tofu, mashed
1 tsp garlic purée
1 tsp tarragon or other dried herbs
Salt or herb salt to taste
Lemon juice to taste
Soya milk, creme or mayonnaise

Mix together, adding enough nut or soya milk, creme or mayonnaise to make it hold together.

tofu quiche

1 pack tofu (250g)
1 cup soya milk
2 tbs flour
Seasoning to taste: herb salt, garlic, yeast flakes
2 cups cooked vegetables

Spread the cooked vegetables in an uncooked pie shell – see recipe below. Whizz the rest of the ingredients in the blender for a few seconds, then pour the mixture over the vegetables in the pie shell. Cook in a moderate oven until the filling becomes solid and the top begins to brown.

wholemeal pastry (with oil)

1 cup whole-wheat flour
1 cup porridge oats
⅓ cup olive oil
½ cup water

Mix thoroughly and roll out on a sheet of cling film or greaseproof paper. It can be used for quiches, pies or crackers. This makes a crispy pastry, suitable for savoury or sweet pies or tarts. It is very easy to mix, but is inclined to break when rolled out, so except for very small things, roll out on cling film or greaseproof paper. For a shiny glaze, brush the top of pies with soya milk before cooking.

12

Depending on how thinly it is rolled out, this recipe should make enough pastry for a 24cm (9½ in) covered pie, or two slightly smaller open tarts.

100% wholefood no oil pastry

1 cup porridge oats
1 cup whole wheat flour
1½ cups sunflower seeds (or nuts), finely ground in blender or coffee mill
½-1 cup water

Mix everything together, roll out and use as for wholemeal pastry.

For a **pre-cooked pie shell**, roll out pastry and line pie dish, pricking the base with a fork. To ensure that the empty pie shell keeps its shape in the oven, fill it with dried beans (that you can keep for this purpose). Bake it for 15-20 minutes in a moderately hot oven.

wholemeal pastry crackers

Roll the pastry out *thinly*, cut into squares or strips and bake it in a moderately hot oven until golden brown (10-15 minutes).

one pot vegetable dishes

These dishes all start in the same way with 1 medium sized onion, rather finely chopped or sliced and gently sautéed with 1 tbs of olive oil. 1-2 crushed garlic cloves are a recommended option. When the onions are transparent, add the rest of the ingredients, put the lid on and leave the vegetables to simmer gently until they are cooked. Seasoning is according to your taste – use stock cubes, herb salt, or just salt. The advantage of these dishes is that as everything is cooked in the same pot together, so all the vegetable juices are conserved. Add some beans or lentils if you would like more protein. Serve with some starch – rice, couscous or potatoes – and you have a complete meal.

A note about oil options

You can use less oil, or more oil or omit the oil completely.

Some recipe suggestions:
Winter mix: onion, celery, carrot, potato, swede, celeriac.

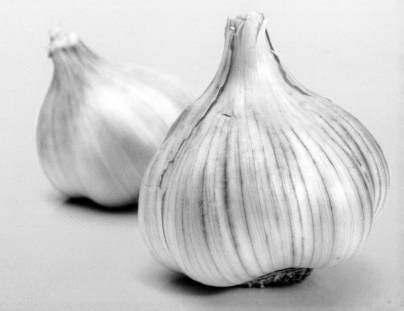

Cabbage mix: onion, rather finely chopped or sliced, sweet pepper, thinly sliced, 3-4 cupfuls of finely sliced cabbage, 2-3 tbs tomato purée or 1 tin chopped tomatoes.

Ratatouille: onion, green or red sweet pepper, 2 or 3 small courgettes, 1 small aubergine, 2-3 tbs tomato purée, bouquet garni or herbes de Provence to taste.

Courgette stew: ratatouille without the aubergine. The courgettes can be sliced, in chunks or coarsely grated. (You can use marrow in the same way.)

Green beans Provençal: to the usual onion base add several cups of fresh or frozen green beans, 2-3 tbs of tomato paste, and enough boiling water to keep it from sticking. Add seasoning, put on the lid and simmer gently until the beans are cooked.

stir-cooked vegetables

This is healthy, because they are cooked very lightly and very quickly in their own juices, so nothing is thrown away. Very little oil need be used, or it can be omitted altogether.

Traditional stir-fry seasonings include grated fresh ginger root, freshly crushed garlic and soy sauce. Just about any vegetable that can be cut in small strips or slices can be used, for example, onions, cabbage, mushrooms, carrot matchsticks, bean shoots, etc. It takes longer to chop the vegetables than to cook them.

Turn the heat up high, put a little oil or water in the bottom of a wok or large deep frying pan. Add the prepared vegetables and seasonings and stir until they begin to soften, You can add pieces of tofu or other 'vegetarian meat', cashew nuts or whatever you like. It only takes a few minutes to cook.

vegetable pies and casseroles

These filling dishes are meals in themselves. Just add salad to complete it.

Vegetable casserole
Pour a *creamy cashew sauce* (see page 125) over lightly-cooked mixed vegetables, e.g. chopped carrots, potatoes, green peas, leeks, in an ovenproof dish. Cook in the oven until the top is golden brown.
Options:
Cover with a layer of mashed potato, or sprinkle with Crunchy crumb topping.

crunchy crumb topping

Mix together equal quantities of brown breadcrumbs and ground nuts or sunflower seeds. Flavour with seasoning salt and your choice of dried herbs.

123

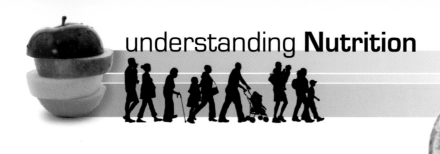

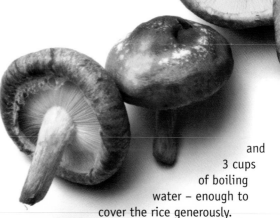

roast potato wedges

(including the skins)
Cut medium sized unpeeled potatoes longways into 4-6 wedges. Steam them until they are almost cooked, then transfer them to a large bowl, containing just enough olive oil to coat them lightly, your choice of seasoning (see below) and salt or herb salt. Mix, put them in a baking tray and cook them in a moderately hot oven until they are golden brown.

Seasoning variations:
Red – add sweet Hungarian paprika
Herb – add rosemary or other dried herbs
Oil and lemon – use citronette salad sauce instead of oil
Oil-free version – use soya milk instead.

risotto and pilaff

These easy rice dishes just need to be served with a large salad to make a complete meal.

risotto

1 medium onion
1 stick celery
1 small green or red pepper
1 clove garlic, crushed
1 tbs olive oil (optional)
1½ cups brown rice
2 tbs tomato purée
½ cup sliced mushrooms
½ cup chopped green olives
½ cup cashews
Herb salt to taste

Chop the first three ingredients and sauté with the olive oil, adding a little water to prevent burning. (Omit this stage for an oil-free version.) Add the rice and tomato purée and 3 cups of boiling water – enough to cover the rice generously. Simmer gently until the rice is cooked, then add the rest of the ingredients, and cook for a few minutes longer. Add a little more water if necessary, as risotto is a moist dish.

pilaff

This is a very easy dry rice dish, and an ideal way to use up leftover cooked rice. It is simply long grain rice mixed with a selection of colorful and tasty small items. It can be oil free, or the onions and other items can be sautéed in a little olive oil.

rice for pilaff

2 cups long grain brown or white rice
5 cups water
Salt or vegetable stock cube to taste
Bay leaf
For a golden pilaff, add ½-¾ tsp turmeric to the cooking water.
For a very special golden pilaff add a pinch of saffron instead of turmeric to the cooking water.

Put the rice, water and seasoning in a saucepan with a well fitting lid. Bring it

124

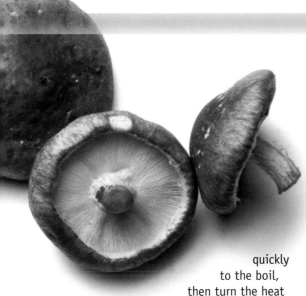

quickly to the boil, then turn the heat right down and let it simmer until all the water is absorbed, about 45-50 minutes for brown rice, 20 for white. The grains should be soft and separate.

Suggested small items to add to rice:
Onion, celery, sweet pepper, green peas, carrot, courgettes, mushrooms, olives, cashews, soya meat chunks, chick peas, sweet corn kernels, artichoke hearts, chestnuts, vegetarian sausages – the larger items cut in fairly small pieces, and the vegetables lightly cooked or raw, according to taste.

Add several cupfuls of items from the list and mix gently with the rice.

The traditional way to serve it is in a large shallow dish and topped with a sprinkling of toasted flaked almonds and raisins.

creamy cashew/sunflower sauce

Basic recipe
3 cups water

½ cup cashews or sunflower seeds (or a mixture)
¼ cup cornflour, barley or other flour
Blend the cashews until smooth in just enough of the water to cover them. Add the cornflour and some more water and blend again before adding the rest of the water. Cook gently for a few minutes, stirring until it thickens. Add more water for a thinner sauce.

Savoury creamy sauce – with herb and onion:
Add a small onion and a clove of garlic while blending, and a handful of fresh parsley, just before turning off the blender. Add herb salt to taste.

Sweet creamy sauce:
Sweeten to taste with honey, apple juice concentrate or maple syrup. Or add a few softened dates. Serve with apple crumble, etc.

white sauce

1 cup soya milk
2 tbs flour
½ tbs oil
Seasoning to taste
Blend thoroughly, pour into saucepan and cook, stirring, for a few minutes until it thickens, then turn down heat and cook for a further few minutes, stirring occasionally. For parsley sauce, add a handful of parsley leaves and ½ small onion to the blender, plus salt or other seasoning to taste.

Oil-free variation:
Instead of oil use 1-2 tbs cashews or sunflower seeds finely ground in coffee mill, and cook as above.

125

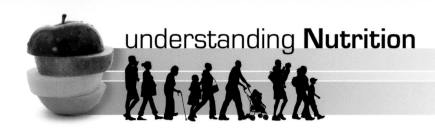
soup suggestions

Soup is good because all the goodness of the ingredients is retained. Thick, filling soups are nourishing, and with bread and salad, you have a whole meal.

cream soups

Dairy-free cream soups can be made with cashew or sunflower cream. Super-easy cream soup is made by cooking everything in the saucepan together, letting it cool briefly, then blending it. For a cream soup with more texture, the cream is made separately and added when the vegetables have cooked. Cashews make the smoothest, richest cream, but sunflower seeds are good too, and are much cheaper, or you can use a mixture of the two.

cream of broccoli (stalk) soup

1 medium sized onion
1 celery stick
1 garlic clove
2 thick broccoli stalks
⅓ cup cashews or sunflower seeds, or a mixture of both
1 vegetable stock cube or other seasoning

Cut the onion, celery and broccoli stalks into a few pieces, and put in a saucepan with the cashews or seeds, and add 1 pint or a generous ½ litre of boiling water. Cover and cook for 15-20 minutes. Allow to cool a little, then blend until smooth. Add more water if desired. Garnish with parsley or fresh chives. For a thicker soup, add a chopped potato, or ¼ cup easy cook white rice before cooking. Or add some left over cooked rice or other cereal before blending.

lentil soup

Basic recipe: 1 medium sized onion, chopped, 1 stick celery, chopped, 1 clove garlic, crushed.

Sauté these with a tbs each of olive oil and water. (Omit this stage for an oil-free version.)

Add 1 cup red lentils, ¼ cup easy cook rice or brown rice flakes plus 1½ pints (scant 900ml) boiling water (add more as needed). Simmer until cooked – about ½ hour.

Season with herb salt or vegetable stock cube and sprinkle with fresh chopped or freeze dried parsley, or fresh coriander leaves.

Variations
Lentil and potato – omit the rice and add 2 cupfuls of chopped potato.
Cabbage – add several cups of rather finely chopped or shredded cabbage.
Cauliflower – add several cups of finely chopped cauliflower.
Tomato – add a 10oz tin of chopped tomatoes or ¼ cup tomato paste.

Seasoning variations
Bouquet garni, oregano, fresh coriander are all very good with this soup, as are ground coriander and cumin, and sweet Hungarian paprika.

120

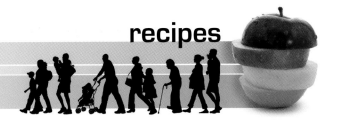

salad – something raw at every meal

Here are some salad suggestions, some plant food alternatives to mayonnaise, and a vinegar-free alternative to vinaigrette. If you want to fill up on highly nutritious, low-calorie foods and leave less room for other things, a big salad is the ideal way to start a meal.

Choose a wide variety of vegetables. These salad recipes are very flexible. Most vegetables can be eaten raw, so the possible variations are enormous. Although most people could eat much more raw food than they do, we do not recommend that you eat all your vegetables raw, as some nutrients are more easily absorbed after cooking. Choose a selection each day, some raw and some cooked, from the wide variety of vegetables that are available now.

Salad dressings are important. They can be as simple as a sprinkling of lemon juice and/or olive oil and salt. Lemon juice aids digestion and oil facilitates the absorption of the fat-soluble vitamins in your salads, so unless you have specific health problems, do not hesitate to use an oil and lemon dressing (in moderation). These dressings are not limited to salads, either: they are very good on baked potatoes and other cooked vegetables. The mayonnaise recipes are for family size quantities, and should keep for 1½-2 weeks in the fridge.

a selection of salads

Tomato salad
Slice tomatoes thinly, arrange on a plate, and sprinkle with French dressing and herbs.

Carrot salad
Finely grate carrot, sprinkle with lemon juice and chopped fresh dill or parsley.

Sweet pepper salad
Slice a sweet pepper thinly, sprinkle with salt and olive oil.

Cucumber salad
For 1 cup of cucumber cut in very thin slices or small cubes (1 cm or less), mix with 1 tbs French dressing, and ½ tbs chopped fresh dill, or ¼ tbs freeze-dried dill.

Tossed salad
The classic tossed salad is made from lettuce or other green leaves with a French dressing. Try lettuce, sliced tomatoes, sliced cucumber, finely sliced onions or chopped chives, and for a dark green colour contrast, some chopped parsley, watercress or rocket.

Winter salad
A classic winter salad is grated carrot and finely shredded white cabbage with French dressing or mayonnaise. Add chopped parsley, chives, dill or other fresh green herbs for

colour and flavour, finely chopped onion for added taste, grated swede for a tang, grated apple for a sweet or tart contrast.

Green, white and orange salad
½ head of Chinese leaf, sliced fairly finely
1 orange, peeled and chopped
Small bunch of dark green leaves such as watercress, rocket, baby spinach, roughly chopped, or parsley, finely chopped.
Mix with 2 tsp olive oil and herb salt to taste.

Carrot and celeriac salad
Grate equal quantities of carrot and celeriac and mix together, with your choice of dressing.

Raw beetroot salad
Mix finely grated raw beetroot with equal parts of grated carrot and apple. Sprinkle with lemon juice and herb salt, or mix with French dressing or mayonnaise, or a mixture of both.

sprinkle toppings for salads
Seeds – sunflower and pumpkin, can be toasted first.
Nuts – chopped or ground walnuts, flaked almonds, cashew pieces, etc.
Olives soothe the digestive system and can be eaten with almost any kind of salad, served separately or mixed in.

sprouted seeds
Mung bean shoots and sprouted alfalfa seeds are probably the best known. Apart from bean shoots, it's not always easy to find them, so if you like them, sprout your own. Sprouted seeds are delicious, and very nutritious too. As the seeds sprout, they develop vitamin C and become more digestible. You can mix them into other salads, or eat them on their own.

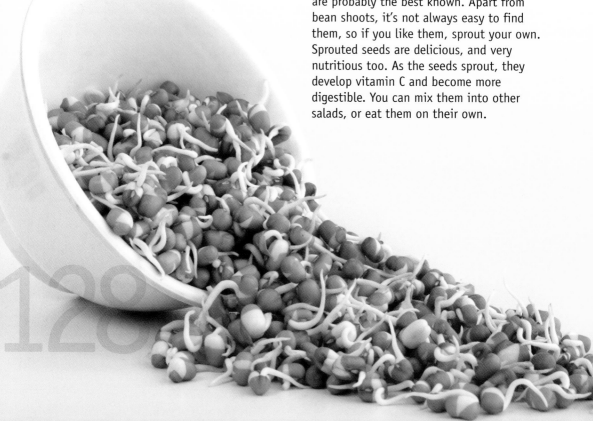

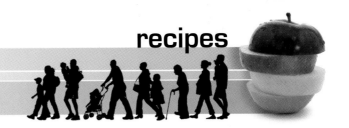

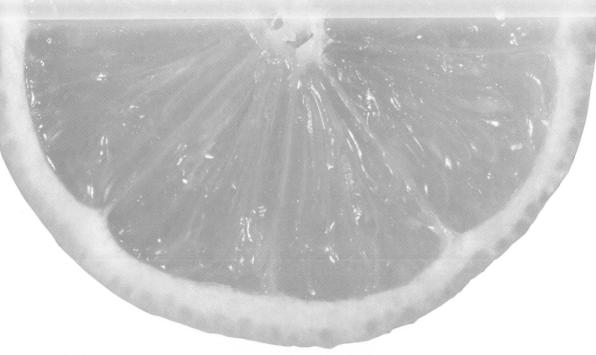

salad dressings
tofu mayonnaise (oil free)

1 250g pack of tofu
½ cup cashews, blended smooth in just enough water to cover
2-3 tbs lemon juice
1 tbs garlic purée, or to taste
Herb salt to taste

Crumble the tofu and add to the blender with the other ingredients and enough soya milk or water to enable the blender blades to turn easily. Blend together briefly. Option – add a handful of fresh parsley with the tofu and other ingredients.

citronette French dressing

¼ cup (or less, according to taste) lemon juice
½ cup olive oil
¼ cup yeast flakes (optional)
1 tbs herb salt, or to taste
1 tbs garlic purée (optional)

Put everything in a jar with a tightly fitting lid, and shake vigorously until thoroughly mixed.

This can be used on cooked vegetables as well as salad, and is excellent with baked potatoes.

It keeps well in the fridge for several weeks.

oil-free citronette

Make exactly as for standard citronette, replacing the oil with soya or any other non-dairy milk, but make in small amounts as it won't keep so well.

129

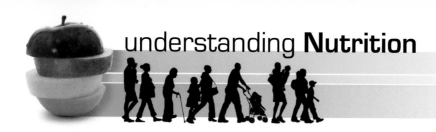
some suggestions for wholefood desserts

100% wholefood no oil sweet pastry for tarts

1 cup porridge oats
1 cup whole wheat flour
1 cup date butter (dates soaked in just enough water to cover)
1½ cups sunflower seeds, ground in blender
½-1 cup water

Mix everything together and roll out, as in previous pastry recipe (page 122).

crunchy granola base for tarts

For an 8 x 10 inch (20 x 25cms) dish, make a pie base with 2 cups granola or crunchy cereal. Grind briefly in blender then mix with 3 tbs water or orange juice and 1 tsp ground coriander. Press mixture over base of dish.

lemon tart

Blend:
3 cups pineapple juice
½ cup orange juice
¼ cup lemon juice
⅓ cup cornflour
⅓-½ cup honey or apple juice concentrate
2 tsp oil (optional)
Grated rind of 1 lemon

Cook over medium heat, stirring until thick, then pour into baked pie shell or onto granola base and cool.

pineapple cream pie

1 cup cashews
3 tbs lemon juice
¼ cup cornflour
1½ cups pineapple juice
2 cups crushed pineapple

Blend the cashews until smooth, in just enough juice to cover them, then blend in everything else except the crushed pineapple. Transfer to a saucepan and cook until it thickens, stirring all the time. Stir in the crushed pineapple and transfer to baked pie shell.

fruit crumble

Apple crumble is the best known, but you can use many different kinds of fruit, or mixtures of fruit.

Traditional fruit crumbles use quite a lot of sugar, but you can use dates, raisins, or apple juice concentrate to sweeten. Here are some suggestions:

Apple and raisin
Rhubarb and date
Plum and blackberry with raisins
Blackcurrant and apple with date

NB: Some fruits, particularly some apples, take longer to cook than the topping does, so partly cook them before you add the crumble topping.

When using dried fruit, to sweeten, use one cup of dried fruit to 2-3 cups

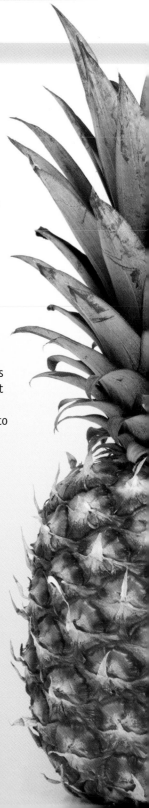

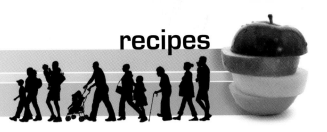
of fresh fruit, depending how sweet the fresh fruit is. Add one cup of water for each cup of dried fruit plus some extra, depending on the size of the crumble. Put the fruit mixture in a fairly shallow baking dish, spread a layer of crumble over the top and cook in a moderately hot oven until the crumble starts to brown and the fruit is cooked.

Crumble topping A

1 cup whole wheat flour
1 cup rolled oats
¼ cup oil
Enough apple juice concentrate or honey to give it a crumbly consistency when mixed together lightly.

Crumble topping B

1 cup porridge oats
1 cup whole wheat flour
1 cup dates soaked in enough water to cover
1½ cups sunflower seeds, ground in blender
Mix it together, adding extra water if necessary, to make it crumbly.

date and coconut cookies

1 cup chopped dried dates, soaked in just enough water to cover them
1 cup sunflower seeds, ground in blender
1 cup desiccated coconut
1 cup rolled oats
½ tsp vanilla essence

Mix all ingredients together well and form into small balls, adding a little water if necessary. Place the cookies on an oiled baking tray and press them flat with a fork. Bake in a moderate oven until they are golden brown, then cool them on a wire rack. Makes 15-20 cookies.

Variations:
You can use any seed, nut, dried fruit or flour, and any fruit juice instead of water.

If you like it extra sweet, add an extra ½ cup of dates, or add 1-2 tbs of apple juice concentrate, runny honey or malt extract. If this makes it too sticky, and a little more oats.

You can use nuts instead of or as well as the coconut or sunflower seeds. Grind nuts in the blender first, or chop them finely.

Try chopped, dried apricots and/or raisins instead of dates, plus liquid to bind it. Apple sauce or mashed banana are two possibilities.

If you like it spicy, add a teaspoonful of coriander seeds and a cardamom pod to the sunflower seeds in the blender.

No blender? The cookies will just be more crumbly and chewy, but some prefer them like that anyway.

Bars: spread the mixture about 2cms thick on an oiled tray, and cut into bars or squares when cooked.

131

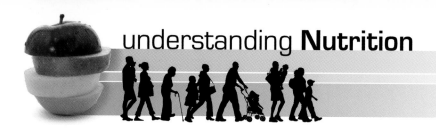
Thin crisp biscuits

The ingredients are the same as for the cookies. If you are using chopped dried dates, rather than softening them in water, grind them finely in the blender. This works best if you grind them with seeds or nuts. Add enough liquid to make a dough that you can roll out thinly, cut into circles or squares and bake in a moderate oven until crisp (10 - 15 minutes). Cool on a wire rack.

peanut butter or tahini flapjack

1 cup peanut butter or tahini
½ cup honey
4 cups rolled oats

Mix together thoroughly, press onto a flat baking tray (e.g. 8 inches or 20cms square). Bake in a moderate oven until firm and golden brown. Cut into squares or bars while still hot.

Cool on tray or wire rack.

smoothies

Smoothies are almost always popular, especially with the young. They are very quick and easy to make, and very versatile. The number of varieties depends only on your imagination and what is available in the shops. They can be as liquid or as solid as you choose to make them – to drink with a straw, or to eat with a spoon like a soft ice-cream. They can also be frozen as ice lollies, or an ice-cream machine can transform them to sorbet or ice-cream.

fruit smoothie

Frozen bananas* cut in small chunks
Fruit juice
Fruit

Use any fruit and any juice. There should be enough juice to cover the bananas in the blender. The other fruit can be fresh (cut in reasonably small pieces), dried – softened (dates) or cooked (apricots, raisins). If berries with small hard seeds are used, the smoothie should be sieved.

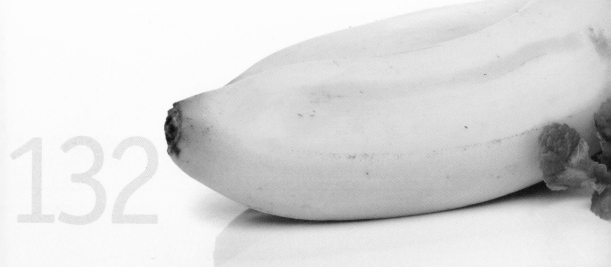

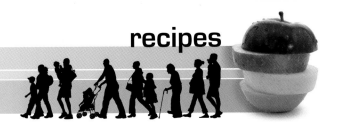

Basic fruit smoothie to start with: frozen banana, orange juice, dried apricots. Sweeten with date, raisins, honey, apple juice concentrate – even sugar – if necessary. Just blend it all together until smooth.

cream smoothie

Frozen bananas* cut in small chunks
The 'cream' can be coconut milk, tofu, soya milk, cashews (be sure to blend them until smooth before adding other ingredients).
Fruit – berries or blackcurrants, lightly cooked, puréed, strained and cooled, or other fruit.
There should always be enough liquid to allow the blender blades to turn easily.

To freeze bananas, remove skins, put in airtight bags or containers and freeze.

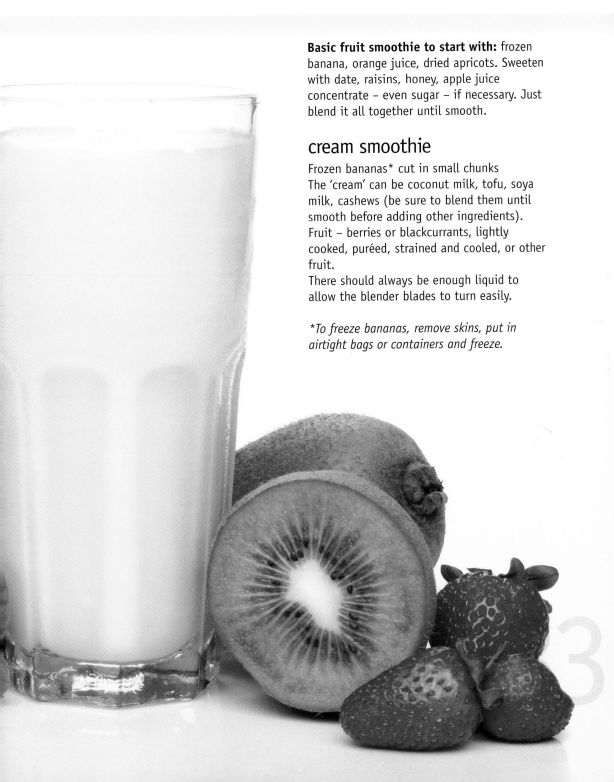

other titles to accompany
understanding **Nutrition**

Want some more recipes?
Then try these little recipe books, also by Dr Clemency Mitchell.

Better Breakfasts
50+ wholefood ideas and recipes to give you the best possible start to your day.

Soups, Salads and Sandwiches
50+ recipes to help you make wholesome, healthy food tasty and tempting.

Desserts and other festive food
60+ recipes for tasty, tantalising desserts and scrumptious festive food.

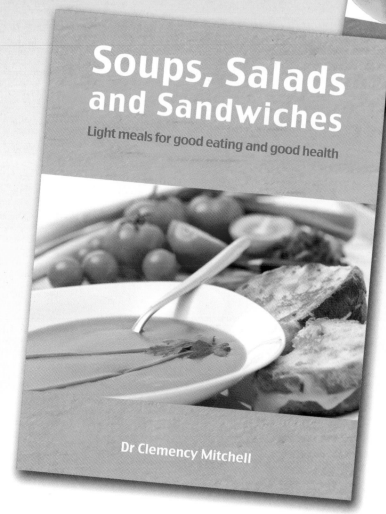

Soups, Salads and Sandwiches
Light meals for good eating and good health

Dr Clemency Mitchell

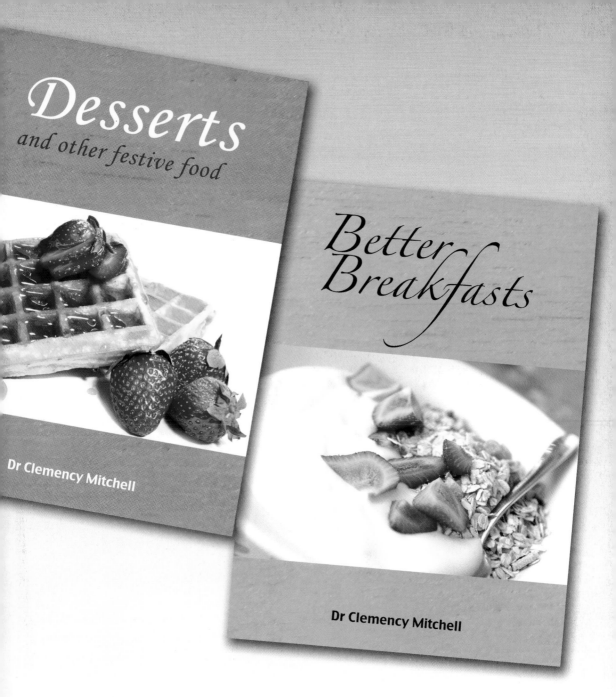

Desserts
and other festive food

Dr Clemency Mitchell

Better
Breakfasts

Dr Clemency Mitchell

All available from your local Adventist Book Centre.